Chronic Pelvic Pain in Women

Edited by M. Renaer

With 22 Figures and 10 Tables

Springer-Verlag
Berlin Heidelberg New York 1981

Marcel Renaer, M. D., Ph. D., F. R. C. O. G., a. e.

Professor and Head
Department of Obstetrics and Gynecology
A. Z. St. Rafael, Kapucijnenvoer 33
3000 Leuven, Belgium

ISBN 3-540-10608-1 Springer-Verlag Berlin Heidelberg New York
ISBN 0-387-10608-1 Springer-Verlag New York Heidelberg Berlin

Library of Congress Cataloging in Publication Data. Main entry under title: Chronic pelvic pain in women. Bibliography: p. Includes index. 1. Pelvis-Diseases. 2. Abdominal pain. 3. Backache. 4. Generative organs, Female-Diseases. I. Renaer, M. [DNLM: 1. Female. 2. Pain. 3. Pelvis. WE 750C557] RG482.C47 617'.55 81-326

Typesetting, printing and bookbinding: G. Appl, Wemding
2125/3140-543210

Preface

The number of studies on chronic and recurrent pain bears no relation to the frequency of these complaints in gynecologic practice, nor to the clinical and scientific problems that still need solving in this area.

Several factors stand in the way of progress in this field, such as the strongly subjective nature of the complaints, the frequent lack of correlation between them and objective findings, and the complexity of the psychosomatic interactions involved.

Although progress in our knowledge has been much slower than we would have wished, and although we are well aware of these many gaps, it was considered useful to gather in a book what we think we have learned during 3 decades of active interest in pain patients and pain problems in gynecologic practice and 12 years of supervision of a pain clinic in the Department of Obstetrics and Gynecology of Leuven University.

As there are many differences between acute pain – clinical as well as experimental – on the one hand and chronic pain symptoms on the other, it was felt preferable to limit the scope of this book essentially to chronic and recurrent pain in gynecologic practice.

When presented with a complaint of lower abdominal and/or low back pain, the gynecologist should constantly be on the lookout for nongynecologic causes, of which the most frequent will be either gastroenterologic or orthopedic and sometimes urologic. I have been fortunate in obtaining the collaboration of Dr. N. C. Hightower of the Department of Gastroenterology and Dr. J. W. Roberts of the Department of General Surgery of the Scott and White Clinic (Temple, Texas, United States), who wrote the extensive review on lower abdominal pain of enterocolic origin. Professor E. Morscher, Professor of Orthopedic Surgery of Basel University (Switzerland), has been kind enough to contribute the chapter on diagnosis and treatment of the orthopedic causes of low back pain. Dr. R. Vereecken, Associate Professor of Urology at Leuven University (Belgium), wrote the survey of the urologic causes of lower abdominal and low back pain and Dr. H. Adriaensen and Prof. J. Gybels (Leuven) the chapter on pain due to gynecologic tumors.

Because of the ubiquity of psychological influences in pain problems, psychological evaluation of the complaints and of the patient's personality should go hand in hand with somatic exploration, which should not just be left to another specialist. Difficult diagnostic and therapeutic problems are so frequently encountered as to regularly necessitate the help of a psychiatrist interested in the psychopathology of everyday life. We have been happy to enjoy, ever since the start of our gynecologic pain clinic, the close collaboration of a psychiatrist in our department. His domain and that of his collaborators – initially psychosomatic gynecology – has steadily expanded and now encompasses (besides marriage and family problems) requests for adoption, for donor insemination, for surgical sterilization, and for abortion. With this experience as a background, our colleague, Prof. P. Nijs (Leuven) kindly undertook to write the chapter on the psychological aspects of chronic pain complaints.

To all these collaborators I extend my heartfelt thanks for the time and energy they invested in the preparation of their contributions.

It is fitting that I express my gratitude to those who initiated me in the problems of chronic pain in gynecology, in particular, Prof. R. Schockaert and Prof. J. A. Schockaert (Leuven), Prof. James Young, British Postgraduate Medical School (Hammersmith, London), and Prof. H. C. Taylor (Columbia Presbyterian Medical Center, New York).

I wish to thank Dr. Phil. Guy A. J. Tops (Universitaire Faculteiten St. Ignatius Antwerpen), who did the linguistic correction of the texts contributed by the Belgian authors. Bernard Shaw would certainly have agreed that writing a book in English with such competent and devoted help is an excellent means of improving one's English.

I also wish to acknowledge my indebtedness to Mrs. Chr. Nijs-Taels, to Mrs. M. Bogaerts-De Messemaecker, and to Mrs. Van Hulst-Toremans for the countless secretarial tasks involved in preparing the manuscript.

My wife will surely be more relieved than anyone else now that "the deed is done."

M. Renaer

Contents

List of Contributors

H. Adriaensen, M. D.
Department of Anesthesiology, University of Leuven, 3000 Leuven, Belgium

J. Gybels, M. D., Ph. D.
Department of Neurology and Neurosurgery, University of Leuven, 3000 Leuven, Belgium

N. C. Hightower, M. D., Ph. D.
Division of Gastroenterology, Scott and White Clinic, Scott and White Memorial Hospital, Temple, TX 76501, USA

E. Morscher, M. D.
Department of Orthopedic Surgery, University of Basle, 4055 Basle, Switzerland

P. Nijs, M. D.
Department of Obstetrics and Gynecology, University of Leuven, 3000 Leuven, Belgium

J. W. Roberts, M. D.
Division of General Surgery, Scott and White Memorial Hospital, Temple, TX 76501, USA

R. L. Vereecken, M. D.
Department of Urology, University of Leuven, 3000 Leuven, Belgium

1 Introduction

Chronic and recurrent lower abdominal or low back pain, together with abnormal bleeding and leukorrhea, ranks among the most common complaints in gynecologic practice. The frequency of the complaint will vary according to certain circumstances. The cultural background of a population influences its readiness to present pain complaints; the special interest of a particular doctor in pain problems will encourage patients to seek his or her counsel, and the known lack of interest of an outpatient clinic will prevent patients from presenting this symptom.

1.1 Frequency of Chronic Pain

If patients consulting for contraception are discounted, it is estimated that about one-fourth of all patients in a nonspecialized gynecologic pratice have some form of chronic or recurrent pain as their main complaint. The high frequency of chronic pain syndromes can be deduced from the numbers of laparoscopies performed for pain in many gynecologic clinics. The Report on the Confidential Enquiry into Gynaecological Laparoscopy (1978) conducted by the Royal College of Obstetricians and Gynaecologists mentions "pain" as a major indication in 51,7% of some 21000 diagnostic laparoscopies. In the Department of Obstetrics and Gynecology of Leuven University, a series of 200 consecutive diagnostic laparoscopies were performed during a 14-month period in 1972 and 1973; chronic pelvic pain was the main reason for performing 108 of these. Clearly, for every patient with chronic pain who is taken into the clinic for exploration and laparoscopy, there are several others for whom a clinical admission is not deemed necessary.

1.2 Frequent Incorrect Diagnoses

Gynecologists and physicians regularly see patients who underwent one or more abdominal operations for a pain condition and still have complaints. The difficulty of diagnosing acute, chronic, or recurrent lower abdominal pain syndromes is clearly revealed in an interesting paper, "Appendicitis in Young Women" (Lee 1961). In a report on 18000 appendectomies performed in clinics of the National Health Service, it was found that 7500 more appendectomies had been performed on young women than on young men between the ages of 14 and 21 (Fig. 1). Yet it has been proved that acute appendicitis is not more common in young women than in young men (Eisele et al. 1956; Green and Watkins 1946). It may be inferred that a high percentage of the appendectomies in young women had been performed on the basis of a wrong diagnosis and that many of the wrongly diagnosed conditions probably had a gynecologic origin, such as dysmenorrhea with a unilateral, right-sided pain localization, unilateral mittelschmerz, and pain due to endometriosis, We will later dwell in detail on the most important causes of erroneous diagnoses.

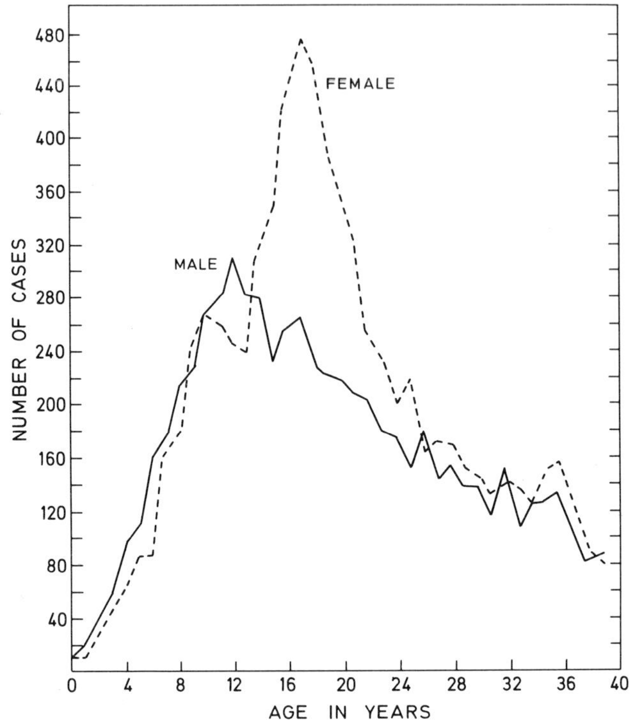

Fig. 1. 18,000 appendectomies performed in clinics of the N.H.S. Lee JA (1961)

1.3 Two-Staged Clinical Investigation of Chronic Pain Syndromes

Examination of patients with lower abdominal pain with or without low back pain generally takes place in two stages. The outpatient clinic separates the cases in whom the diagnosis is clear and who can be treated on an outpatient basis from those who will require a complete work-up.

Several years ago, we noted the origin of the pain in a series of 100 consecutive patients who consulted mainly for chronic or recurrent pain at our gynecologic outpatient clinic. As the diagnoses were based on clinical examinations only, they were essentially probability diagnoses. In 52 patients the pain was felt to have a gynecologic origin, in 24 it had no gynecologic origin, and in another 24 it was considered to have a combined origin. This superficial screening shows that women tend to ascribe lower abdominal and low back pain to gynecologic causes although it may just as well have an orthopedic, a gastrointestinal, or a parietal origin. It also draws attention to the fact, already pointed out by Martius in 1939, that chronic pain complaints frequently have a combined origin; in other words, that the pain may in part be due to a gynecologic and in part to an orthopedic or a gastroenterologic or some other cause.

When the diagnosis is not clear or when the attempted treatment has been of no avail, a complete work-up, which will generally include a laparoscopy, is indicated.

Table 1. Final diagnosis after laparoscopy in 108 consecutive patients with chronic pain as their main symptom

Chronic pelvic pain without obvious pathology	28
Endometriosis	22
"Chronic salpingitis"	23
Various	35
Cause unclear	12
Pain of combined origin	8
Gastroenterologic origin	5
Psychogenic origin	2
Pelvic cellulitis	2
Urologic origin	2
Miscellaneous	4

Table 1 gives the conclusion arrived at after a diagnostic work-up in the 108 cases with chronic pain of a series of 200 consecutive laparoscopies.

Table 1 does not give the full list of all possible causes of chronic and recurrent pain in gynecologic practice. For example, dysmenorrhea, mittelschmerz, and displacement of genital organs are not mentioned as they generally do not necessitate a laparoscopy. Cases of orthopedic pain diagnosed at the outpatient clinic are referred to the orthopedist. Even after a complete clinical investigation the case may remain obscure, as in 12 of the 108 in Table 1. Only two cases of psychogenic pain are mentioned, but they are not at all suggestive of the real importance of psychological factors. In Chap. on 18, it will be shown that there are many reasons for assigning an important role to psychological influences in the pathogenesis of this syndrome.

References

Eisele CW, Slee VW, Hoffmann RG (1956) Can the practice of internal medicine be evaluated? Ann Intern Med 44:144–160

Green HW, Watkins V (1946) Appendicitis in Cleveland; final report. Surg Gynecol Obstet 83:613–624

Lee JA (1961) Appendicitis in young women. Lancet II:815–817

Martius H (1939) Die Kreuzschmerzen der Frau. Thieme Leipzig

Report on the Confidential Enquiry in Gynaecological Laparoscopy (1978) Royal College of Obstetricians and Gynaecologists, London

2 Anatomy and Physiology of Gynecologic Pain

2.1 Innervation

The lower abdominal wall and the anterior part of the vulva are innervated by mixed (motor and sensory) nerves originating from the ventral branches of L-1 and L-2, i. e., the ilioinguinal, the iliohypogastric, and the genitocrural nerves. Dorsal rami derived from L-1 and L-2 (superior clunial nerves) innervate the region of the lower back, where pain sensations due to gynecologic causes are felt.

Impluses originating in the perineum and the lower part of the vagina are conveyed by branches of the pudendal nerves, which are themselves derived from S-2, S-3, S-4 (see Fig. 2a, b)

Noxious impulses from the corpus uteri, the medial part of the fallopian tubes, the cervix, and the upper part of the vagina travel by way of visceral afferents that accompany the sympathetic nerves of the uterus and enter the spinal cord at T-11, T-12, and L-1. When leaving the uterus these visceral afferents travel through the inferior hypogastric – or uterovaginal – plexus, the hypogastric nerves, the superior hypogastric plexus, and the lumbar and lower thoracic sympathetic chain (Fig. 3). Then they pass through the proximal part of the spinal nerves and their posterior roots and make synoptic connections with neurons in the posterolateral tract of Lissauer and the dorsal horn, where the impulses are subjected to various modulating influences. Part of the impulses that are transmitted pass cephalad through the spinothalamic pathways and thence to the sensory cortex.

It has long been thought that the nociceptive impulses from the cervix were conveyed to the sacral segments (S-2, S-3, S-4) of the spinal cord via the pelvic nerves or nervi erigentes. However, Bonica (1953) has shown that nociceptive impulses from the cervix, the body of the uterus, and the adnexa are transmitted through afferent fibers that accompany the above-mentioned sympathetic nerves and that there is no evidence for an afferent pain pathway from the uterine cervix to the sacral segments.

Nociceptive impulses are transmitted from the pelvic walls and the genital organs to the neuraxis via A and C fibers associated with somatic and visceral nerves. Somatic nociceptives fibers are those that supply skin, muscles, bones and joints, and parietal peritoneum, while those that supply the internal genital organs are visceral nociceptive fibers. The lesser sensitivity of most visceral organs compared to superficial somatic structures seems to be due to the lower number of sensory fibers in the visceral nerves.

2.2 Central Pathways and Modulating Influences

Conscious awareness of pain depends on nociceptive impulses that reach the sensory cortex. Somatic structures, such as the right hand and the tongue have well-defined projections in the cortex; impulses of visceral origin mainly ascend in the central nervous system via the indirect spinothalamic or spino-

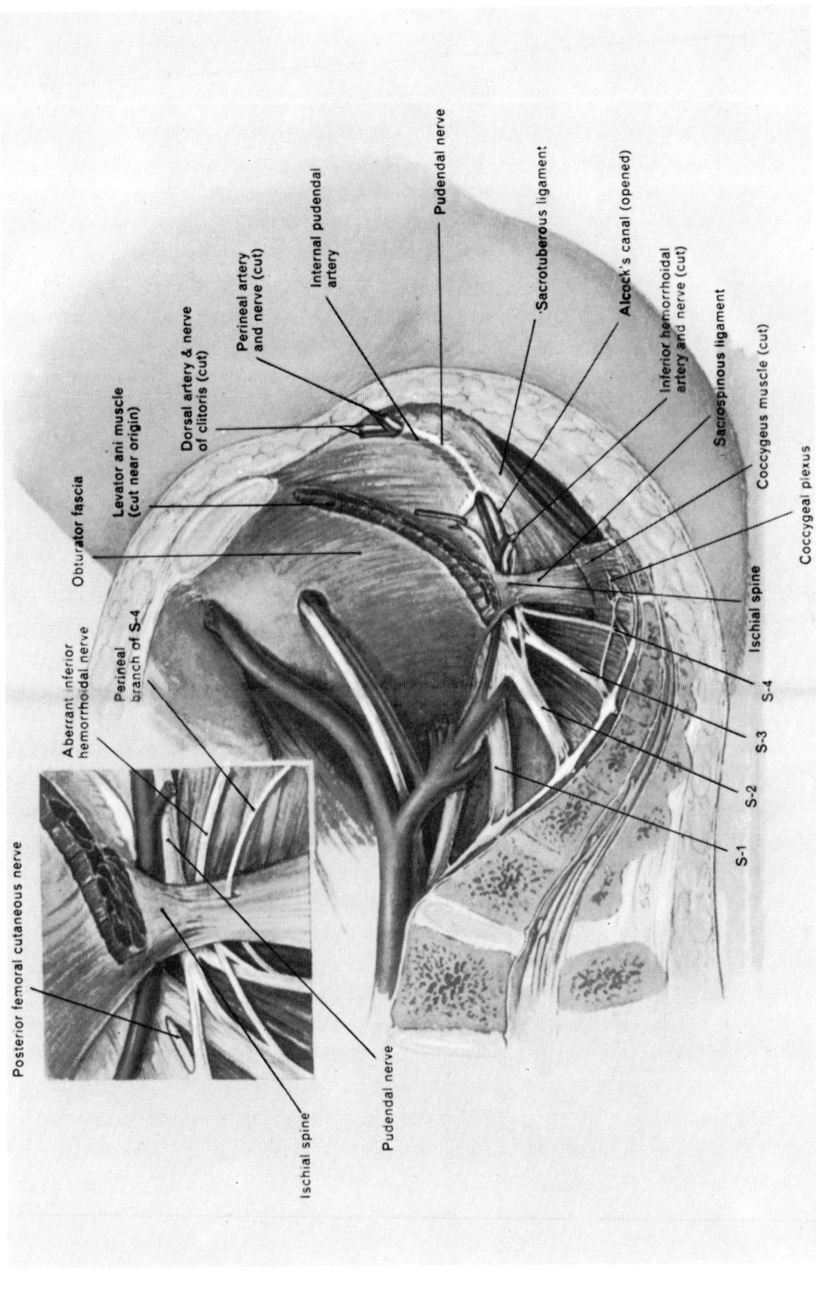

Fig. 2. a Sacral plexus; pudendal and perineal nerves

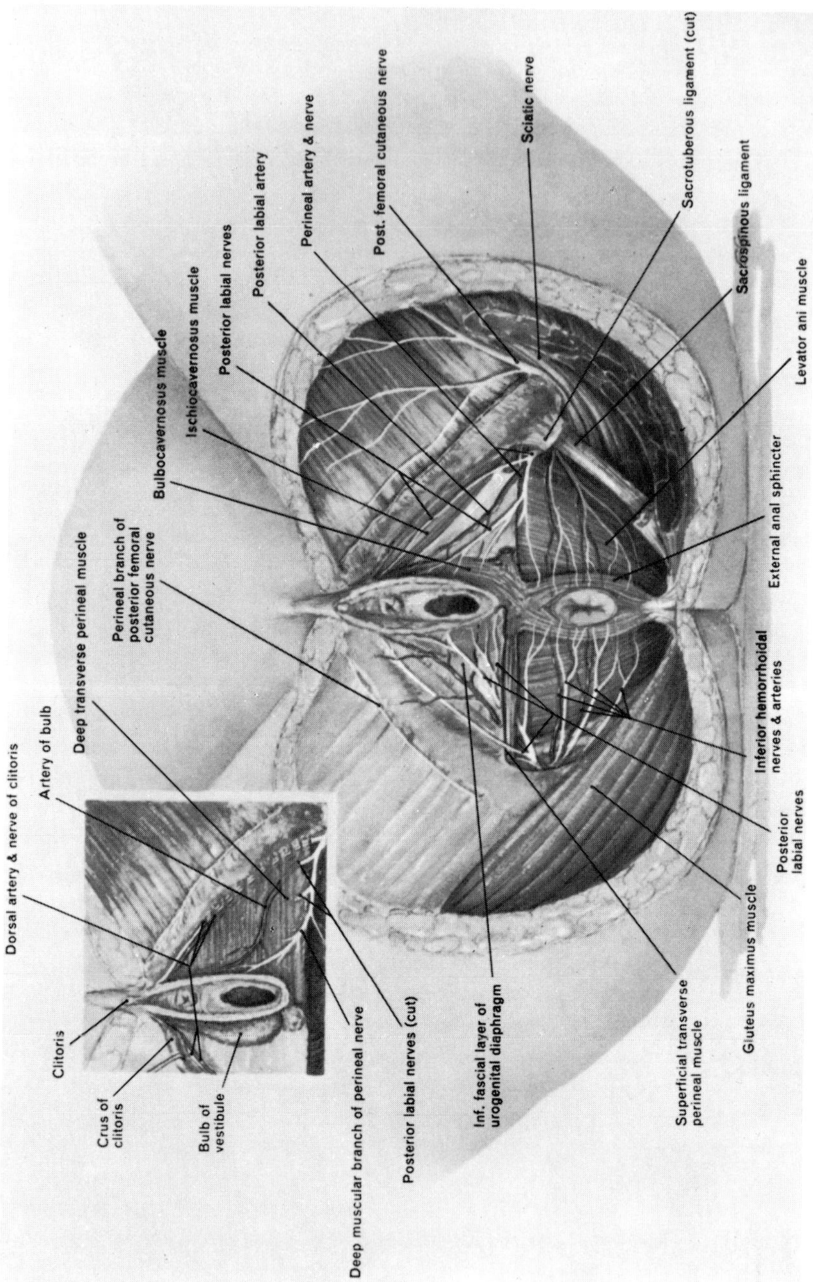

Fig. 2. b Innervation of the external female genitalia. Bonica (1960)

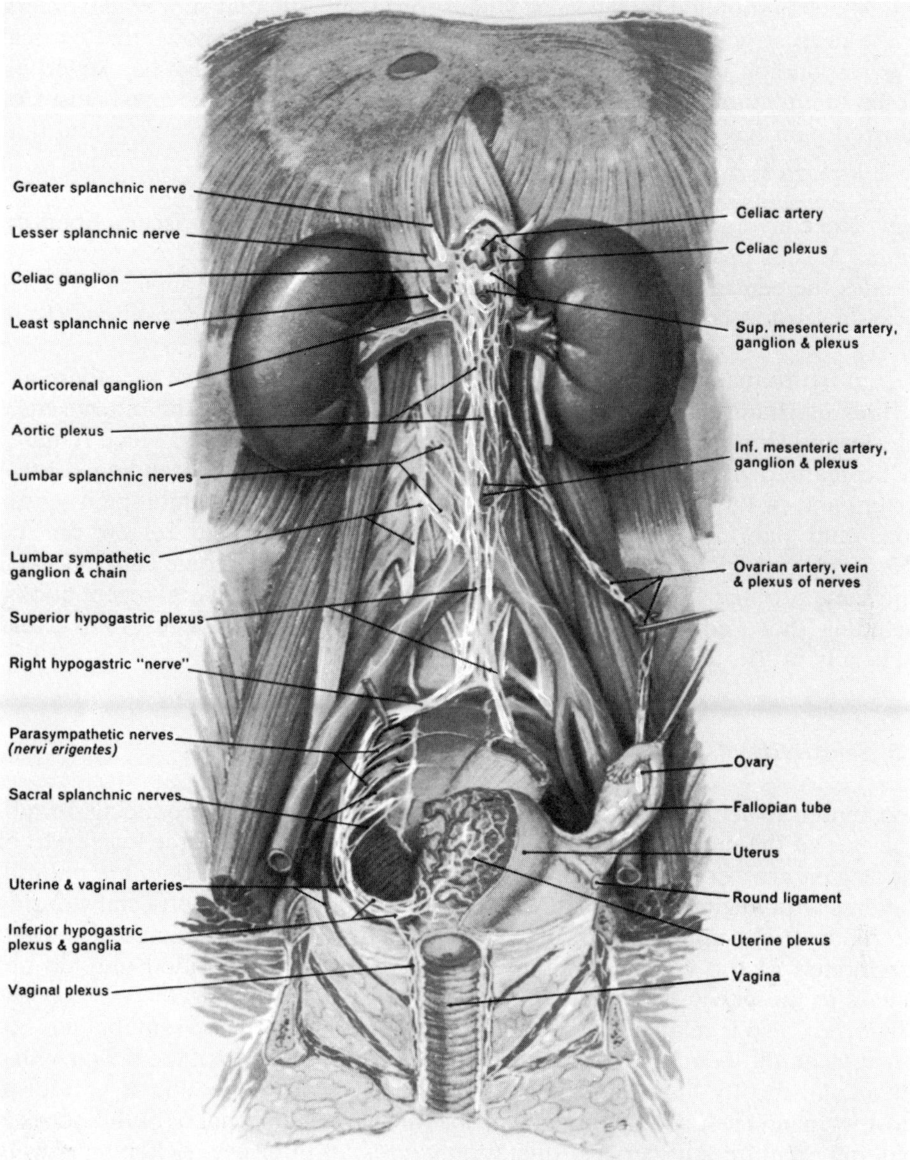

Fig. 3. Innervation of the internal female genitalia. Bonica (1960)

reticulothalamic pathway. They also reach localized areas in the cerebral cortex (Newman 1974), but they have no such differentiated cortical representation as somatic structures so that for a particular visceral organ no corresponding cortical projection can be found.

Visceral pain and pain from deep somatic structures generally has a less accurate, more diffuse, localization than somatic pain. Both are often referred to the skin, which is supplied by the same spinal cord segments that supply the viscera or the deep structures (referred pain). Newman (1974) has shown that cortical cells responding to stimulation of the splanchnic nerve can also be excited by tactile stimulation applied to the skin of the same side. The mechanism of referred pain has been elucidated by Pomeranz et al. (1968), who found that cells located in lamina V (Rexed) of the posterior horn of the cat respond both to fine myelinated afferents from the splanchnic nerve and to afferents from the skin. The convergence of impulses conveyed by cutaneous and visceral fibers on lamina V cells probably explains referred pain.

Besides the central afferent pathway just described, there are apparently other ascending tracts conveying impulses, which may lead to pain sensations (Kerr 1975).

Recent neuroanatomic and neurophysiologic research has shown that there are various mechanisms that modulate, either in an excitatory or inhibitory sense, the sensory stimuli transmitted from the periphery to the brain. Much remains to be learned in this field. A concise description of the descending control system and of the psychological factors that may enhance or inhibit pain sensations and pain reactions may be found in Bonica's lucid review on the "Neurophysiologic and Pathologic Aspects of Acute and Chronic Pain" (1977). The same problems have been treated more extensively in several recent books, including those edited by Hill (1976), Lipton (1977), and Lee (1977); and especially in *The Psychology of Pain* by Sternbach (1978).

2.3 Sensitivity of the Genital Organs

The genital structures are sensitive in varying degrees to pain-producing stimuli. The skin of the perineum and the mucosae of the vulva and of the lower part of the vagina are very sensitive; perineal injuries and scars can be quite painful. Patients with vaginitis may complain of burning or "rawness" especially during intercourse. The upper part of the vagina is relatively insensitive, and ulcers and carcinomas of the vagina generally do not cause pain, provided they do not extend to the pelvic side wall.

The cervix also is relatively insensitive. It can, however, not be said that it is not sensitive at all. Indeed, clamping the anterior or posterior lip of the cervix with a tenaculum mostly hurts, and performing an electrocauterization is painful in most women. The introduction of a probe through the internal os of the cervix is generally painful and cervical dilatation causes an intensive, sickening pain in the depth of the pelvis. This seems to be due to a great density of nerve terminals around the internal os (Keiffer 1935, 1936). Taking a biopsy of the endometrium is less painful. The uterine corpus is less sensitive than the isthmus, probably because the innervation is richer at the isthmus and sparser at the fundus. Under certain circumstances uterine contractions may give rise to pain, but under other circumstances very strong contractions may remain painless (Eskes 1978, personal communication). There are reasons to assume that uterine contractions are especially painful when pressure is exerted by uterine contents on nerve endings at the level of the internal os, as in dysmenorrhea, during a miscarriage, and during labor.

Ovaries are insensitive to many stimuli but are sensitive to others, such as squeezing during bimanual examination. Distension of the ovarian parenchyma by a slowly developing ovarian cyst is not painful, but clinical observation tends to show that more rapid distension of the parenchyma may give rise to pain. The fallopian tube is sensitive to cutting, crushing, and touching (Jeffcoate 1975).

References

Bonica JJ (1953) The management of pain. Lea & Febiger, Philadelphia Pa
Bonica JJ (1960) Whats new, vol 217. Abbott, Chicago, p 16
Bonica JJ (1977) Neurophysiologic and pathologic aspects of acute and chronic pain. Arch Surg 112:750–761
Hill O (1976) Modern trends in psychosomatic medicine – 3. Butterworths, London
Jeffcoate N (1975) Principles of gynaecology. Butterworths, London
Keiffer H (1935) La structure nerveuse du col utérin chez la femme. Bull Acad R Méd Belg 15:581–588
Keiffer H (1936) Physiologie du systéme nerveux de la femme. In: Binet A, Colaneri X: La douleur en gynécologie. 90–106. L'Expansion Scientifique Française, Paris
Kerr FWL (1975) Neuro-anatomical substrates of nociception in the spinal cord. Pain 1:325–356
Lee FF (1977) Pain management. Williams & Wilkins, Baltimore
Lipton S (1977) Persistent pain: Modern methods of treatment, vol 1. Academic Press, London
Newman P (1974) Visceral afferent functions of the nervous system. Arnold, London
Pomeranz B, Wall PD, Weber WV (1968) Cord cells responding to fine myelinated afferents from viscera, muscle and skin. J Physiol (Lond) 199:511–532
Sternbach RA (1978) The psychology of pain. Raven, New York

3 General Characteristics of Chronic Pain of Gynecologic Origin

In every field of clinical medicine, pain symptoms are a valuable aid in establishing a diagnosis. The value of these symptoms depends on the care taken in analyzing their characteristics. Indeed, pain analysis constitutes a pointer toward the diagnosis (Lewis 1942; Janzen 1966).

The characteristics described in this chapter essentially concern chronic pain syndromes that are directly due to a gynecologic lesion or cause. There are, indeed, pain syndromes that are only indirectly due to a gynecologic cause and whose characteristics are not amenable to systematization.

The data that follow are derived from the study of some 80 patients in whom chronic pain was certainly or most probably due to a definite gynecologic lesion. The localization and nature of the lesions were verified by laparoscopy or laparotomy (Schockaert and Renaer 1954). The data are thus based on anatomicoclinical correlations and not on any current theory about pain mechanisms. Any such theory should, instead, try to explain these clinical data. The following characteristics will be described:

1) The most frequent localizations of chronic pain of gynecologic origin
2) The radiation or spread of the pain
3) The time-intensity relationship during the menstrual cycle
4) Hyperalgesia of the abdominal wall and of the back in chronic pain syndromes
5) Other useful data

3.1 Most Frequent Localizations

By the term "localizations" we mean direct and not indirect localizations. Examples of indirect localizations of pain of gynecologic origin are pain felt at the level of the diaphragm when its peripheral part is irritated by the hemoperitoneum of an ectopic pregnancy and referred shoulder pain due to irritation of the central part of the diaphragm. Another example is ischialgic pain caused by a stage III or IV carcinoma of the cervix extending to the ischiatic nerve. When the pain-provoking lesion or condition is situated in the pelvis, pains that have a direct gynecologic origin are felt in a ventral or a dorsal zone, or in both zones. These zones are shown in Fig. 4.

The ventral zone is about 8–10 cm high; generally, it does not extend higher than the level of the anterior and superior iliac spines. The dorsal zone also has a height of 8–10 cm. It is localized over the superior half of the sacrum and extends laterally into the gluteal regions. This zone may also be called the superior sacrogluteal zone. Pains originating in the uterus, in the cervix, in the parametria, and generally also painful conditions of the tubes and ovaries may be felt in both these zones. The pain may of course also be felt in a part of them, e. g., in the right or in the left iliac fossa. It will most frequently be felt ventrally, but it may also be felt ventrally and dorsally, and even, though rather infrequently, in the dorsal zone only.

Pain sensations of gynecologic origin (e. g., in some cases of deep-seated pelvic endometriosis) may sometimes be localized at the level of the lower half of the sacrum. Pains originating in the tubes or ovaries may sometimes be felt immediately above the ventral zone, or above the dorsal zone, as shown in Fig. 5.

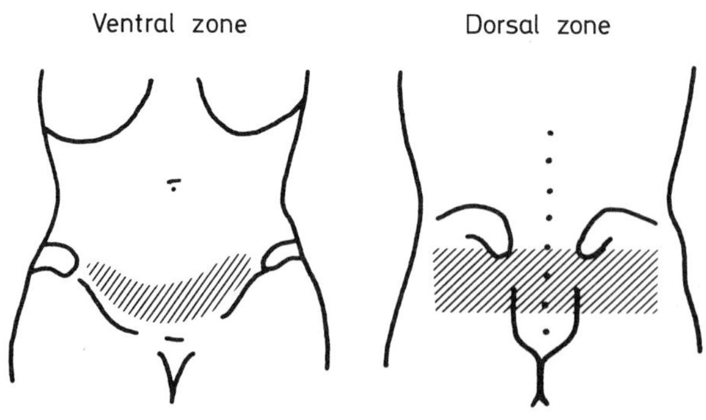

Fig. 4. Usual localizations of chronic pain of gynecologic origin. Renaer (1971) Chronische pijn in de gynaecologische praktijk. Stafleu, Leiden

Of course, the above description of the usual localizations of gynecologic pain brings nothing new, but we have found drawing attention to them useful for two reasons:

1) Chronic pain conditions in which the pain originates in the *internal genital organs* should not be thought of as having vague localizations. While recording the pain complaints, one should therefore be as precise as possible; it is useful to enter into the clinical file a scheme of the localization of the pain.

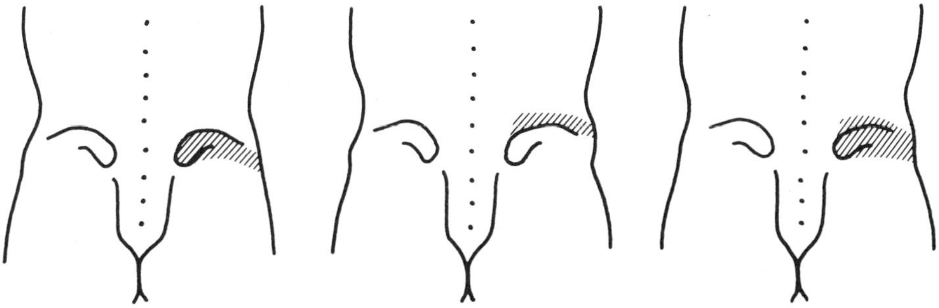

Fig. 5. Infrequent dorsal localizations of pain sensations originating in the adnexa. Renaer (1971) Chronische pijn in de gynaecologische praktijk. Stafleu, Leiden

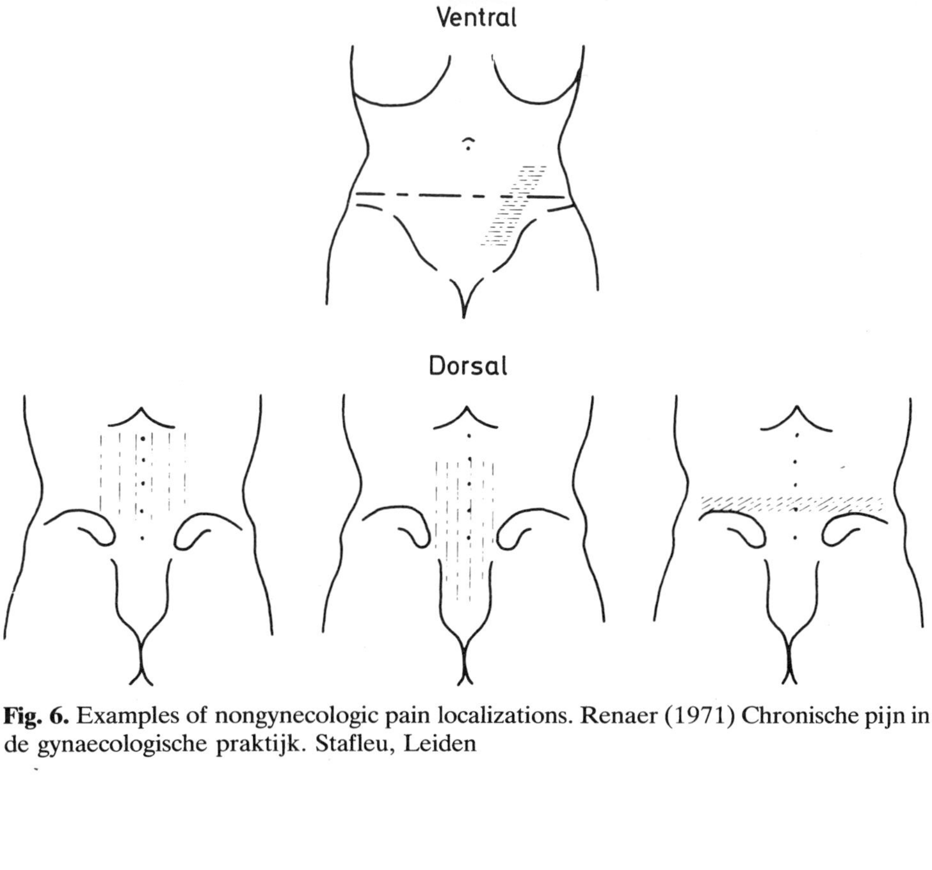

Fig. 6. Examples of nongynecologic pain localizations. Renaer (1971) Chronische pijn in de gynaecologische praktijk. Stafleu, Leiden

To describe dorsal pain, the term "low back pain" is too vague; low backache may indeed be either lumbar, low lumbar, lumbosacral, high sacral, high sacrogluteal, or low sacral, etc. To be able to specify the exact site of the pain, it is necessary to locate it in relation to the vertebral column and to the bony pelvis.

2) The pain zones described above are especially important in a *negative sense.* If the pain sensation is not situated at the level of these zones or if it starts in one of the zones and spreads toward a higher level, it has most probably no gynecologic or at least no direct gynecologic origin (unless the pain is due to a complication of a huge tumor rising well above the pelvic cavity).

Figure 6 gives a few examples of pain localizations that almost certainly have no gynecologic origin.
Lumbar, lumbosacral, and low lumbar pains mostly have an orthophedic origin. Rather infrequently, a patient may not refer her pain to the ventral or the dorsal parietal zones, but experience it in the depth of the pelvis "somewhere midway between those zones." This may happen in some cases of endometriosis. In other instances, the pain localization may be related to the perineum and felt, for example, some 10 cm above the anus, where it can indeed be reproduced by rectal examination.

3.2 Radiation or Spread of Pain

Patients with chronic pain in the lower abdomen may also complain of pain at a higher level of the abdomen or of pain in one or both lower limbs. This may be due either to two different pain localizations or to a propagated pain; both phenomena may have several causes:

1) A *second localization* or a propagation higher up in the abdomen or back should not be attributed to a reflex phenomenon provoked by a gynecologic condition, nor should it be considered as a referred pain due to a gynecologic cause. In fact, the higher pain localization or the upward radiation most probably has no gynecologic origin, or at any rate, no direct gynecologic origin. The second pain localization may be due to a coincidence of, e. g., a painful endometriotic lesion and a functional enterocolopathy. The upward radiation may indirectly have a gynecologic origin, e. g., a subocclusion of the descending colon due to an infiltrating left ovarian carcinoma.
2) If a *pain starting in the lower abdomen* or in the lower back projects into one or both lower limbs, this projection may also be due to various causes; for example, invasion of the sacral plexus by a stage III or IV carcinoma of the cervix will provoke an ischialgic pain. This is an example of an indirect gynecologic pain radiation. Another example would be the rare case in which an endometriotic lesion invades the sacral plexus or the obturator nerve.

Painful conditions of uterine origin, however, such as essential dysmenorrhea or adenomyosis, may give pain projections of variable extension to the anterior part of the thigh. Such pain projections – or referred pains – will be found almost only in the anterior aspect of the thigh, rarely along the inner or outer aspects, and never in the posterior part.

For practical purposes, it follows that an ischialgic pain not due to an invasion of the sacral plexus or of the sciatic nerve by a carcinoma or an endometriosis has no gynecologic origin. Indeed, an ischialgic pain is practically never due to a compression of the plexus or the nerve by a benign gynecologic tumor, even if it is incarcerated in the pelvis; it will only very rarely be due to pressure from an engaged fetal head at the end of pregnancy.

3.3 Time-Intensity Relationship During the Menstrual Cycle

In the majority of chronic painful conditions of gynecologic origin, the history reveals pain fluctuations during the menstrual cycle. In some cases, as in midcycle pain, the time of appearance is characteristic. A pain that gradually becomes more severe toward the end of the menstrual period is suggestive of endometriosis. In other cases, e. g., in posterior pelvic cellulitis or in the so-called pelvic congestion and fibrosis syndrome, the pain becomes more intense in the premenstrual period and diminishes or disappears in the beginning of menstruation. It should, however, be stressed that pains of orthopedic or gastrointestinal origin may also show premenstrual and menstrual exacerbations.

3.4 Hyperalgesia of the Abdominal Wall and of Back in Chronic Pain Syndromes

We have examined the sensitivity of the abdominal wall and of the lower back in many patients with chronic pain of gynecologic origin. When rather heavy pressure is applied with the fingertips on the stretched abdominal wall or on the back, this pressure may, under normal circumstances, cause some discomfort but will not provoke pain. We say that there is "hyperalgesia" if the said stimulus gives rise to pain. It should be remarked that the term "hyperalgesia" as used here does not have the same meaning as in neurology and in pain physiology. To search for this kind of hyperalgesia, the patient should stretch the abdominal wall. She can be instructed to do so either by the technique of Carnett (1926) or by that of Joossens (Renaer and Joossens 1957), which is easier to explain.

As is shown in Fig. 7, the examiner stands at the right side of the patient, who is lying in the supine position. The patient's knees are held down by the left arm of the examiner, and the patient is asked to sit up without using her elbows. While the abdominal wall is stretched, the right hand of the examiner exerts a rather heavy pressure on the site were the pain is localized. With this technique, no pressure is exerted on the abdominal contents. This test does not elicit pain in the normal abdominal wall. In women with chronic pain of gynecologic origin, we almost never found a hyperalgesia of the abdominal wall or of the back as long as the painful condition did not involve the abdominal wall itself or as long as there was no painful condition of the back. We therefore assume that the presence of a hyperalgesia of the abdominal wall or of the back means that the painful condition is in the abdominal wall or in the back itself. Parietal pains in the lower abdomen do not seem to be frequent – they are more freqent in the

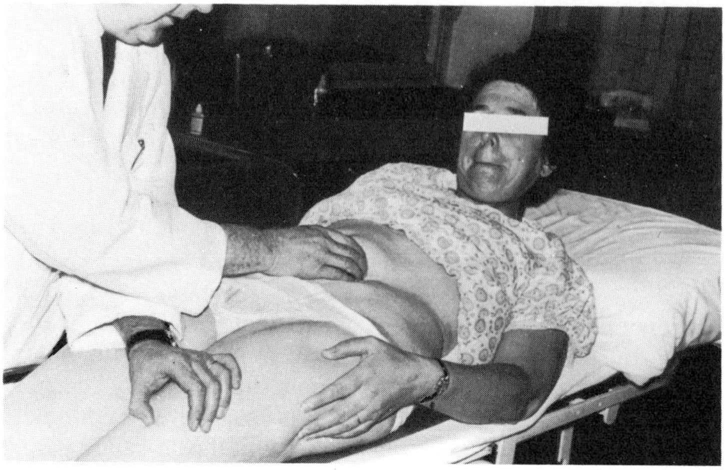

Fig. 7. Looking for hyperalgesia of the abdominal wall. Renaer M (1973) Gynäkologische Schmerzursachen. Der Gynäkologe, vol 6, issue 3:98

back – but as they do occur, one should look for parietal tenderness and pain in every patient who complains of lower abdominal pain and low back pain.

3.5 Other Useful Data

The coincidence of a ventral and a dorsal localization suggests an intrapelvic painful condition. When the pain is felt in the lower back and not in the lower abdomen, it most probably has no gynecologic origin. We certainly agree with the opinion of many orthopedic surgeons that 85% of all cases of low back pain are of orthopedic or rheumatologic origin, although it would seem preferable to say "85% of all cases with low back pain and only low back pain . . ." In his outstanding book *Backache,* Macnab (1977) states that gynecologic disorders rarely (perhaps never) cause low back pain. We concur with this conclusion; indeed, low backache (only) rarely has a gynecologic origin, although in this field, as in many others, one should never say never. Most chronic pains are alleviated by rest. Horizontal rest generally relieves gynecologic pain, but orthopedic pains are alleviated by specific attitudes. Back pains that start during rest and are relieved by movements are apt to be due to a degenerative discopathy. It is well-known that pains due to osseous metastases are relieved neither by rest nor by movements (Morscher 1973). A start pain in the morning is rather characteristic of orthopedic and rheumatic conditions; in these conditions, the pain may also increase with certain movements. This is much less so with gynecologic pain, which will worsen by increased intraperitoneal pressure and by jolts, whereas movements of the trunk do not worsen it.

Painful gynecologic conditions never give rise to rigidity of the vertebral column; such a rigidity will, instead, point toward an othopedic or rheumatologic diagnosis.

It seemed preferable first to describe the characteristics of pain of gynecologic origin before going on to details about history and examination of the patient because these characteristics have in our experience proved very useful as guidelines for the examination of the patient.

References

Carnett JB (1926) Intercostal neuralgia as a cause of abdominal pain and tenderness. Surg Gynecol Obstet 42:625–632

Janzen R (1966) Schmerzanalyse als Wegweiser zur Diagnose. Thieme, Stuttgart

Lewis T (1942) Pain. Macmillan, New York

Macnab I (1977) Backache. Williams & Wilkins, Baltimore

Morscher E (1973) Orthopädisch bedingte Ursachen chronischer Kreuzschmerzen der Frau. Gynaekologe 6:129–133

Renaer M, Joossens JV (1957) Theoretische en praktische beschouwingen over pariëtale pijn (Theoretical and practical thoughts on parietal pain). Verh Vlaamse Akad Geneesk België 19:55–73

Schockaert JA, Renaer M (1954) Contributions à l'étude de la douleur dans la pratique gynécologique. Bull Soc R Belge Gynécol Obstet 24:1–22

4 Examination of Patients with Chronic Pain Syndromes

The purpose of the examination is the collection of data to allow an analysis of the pain sensation and to obtain an integrated view of the patients' pain experience. Some comments will be made on:

1) The patient and her complaints
2) Clinical examination and some special explorations
3) Gynecologic laparoscopy
4) Interpretation of the data

4.1 The Patient and Her Complaints

As we saw earlier, there are several factors that may make a patient decide to present a pain complaint to a doctor. Among them are the intensity of her pain and her emotional reaction toward it. This reaction depends on many circumstances; for example, the meaning or supposed meaning of the pain, the personal history of the patient, her social and cultural environment, the situation in which the pain develops (depression, search for compensation, craving for tenderness, etc.).

As an individual's behavior is to a large extent influenced by environment and heredity, the *family history* may be important in the evaluation of the complaint.

The *personal history* will indicate whether it is the first time the patient consults a doctor or whether this is a particular episode out of a series of ailments. Is there any other pain localization besides the main pain complaint? Is there any other localized or generalized discomfort? Did the present condition begin recently or has it existed for some time, and if it is chronic, what were the earlier diagnoses and treatments and their results? It is also important to know the patient's own opinion about her pain and her attitude toward it. Is she afraid that it may be due to cancer or that it may lead to chronic disablement?

A general practitioner who has been the family doctor of the patient for some time will know the answers to many of these questions. If there is no urgency, the necessary data may be collected by proceeding along a spiral: history taking, examination, evaluation of the data, more inquiry about the complaints and into personal and environmental circumstances, more objective data, reevaluation, etc. We should think more in terms of pain patients than of pain causes (Sternbach 1974).

Many patients with chronic pain have several complaints and frequently seem to behave neurotically. To make things more complicated, several authors have recently shown that one of the effects of chronic pain is emotional instability (Woodforde and Merskey 1972; Sternbach 1974), After a study of the literature and of many personal cases, Merskey (1974, personal communication) states.

> If it is assumed by definition that the group with chronic pain not due to organic causes is neurotic – and this is confirmed by the psychological test scores – then the similar scores of the patients with organic lesions suggest that they are indistinguishable from the psychiatric group in this respect.

4.2 Clinical Examination and Some Special Explorations

4.2.1 History of the Present Disorder

A precise description of the symptoms and signs is needed. No amount of radiologic or laboratory data can replace a careful history, a detailed description of the pain, and a meticulous clinical examination.

The patient should *localize* her pain according to topographical regions or bony landmarks. It is useful to inquire about the localization on different occasions, as visceral or deep pains are nor always easy to localize and a variable localization may point to psychogenic influences.

As explained in Chap. 3, the spread or *radiation* of the pain is equally important as are the circumstances in which the pain started, its duration, and the factors that influence its intensity, such as the activities of the patient, rest or fatigue, bowel functions, the menstrual cycle, emotional turmoil.

Depending on its cause, the pain may begin suddenly, as for example in lithiasis of the kidney or the ureter, or progressively, worsening intermittently, as in many cases of endometriosis. The beginning of the pain may be related to a delivery or a miscarriage (infectious process?), to an operation (parietal pain? adhesions?), or to an emotionally disturbing event. The *nature* of the pain sensation may be useful. Hypogastric cramps will point to the uterus, subumbilical cramps or left flank and left iliac fossa cramps to an enterocolic origin.

Disorders of the internal genital organs may give rise either to shooting pains, to a dull pain, or to a sensation of heaviness or bearing down. A burning pain in the vagina points to a severe vaginitis, but a burning pain or a sensation of something crawling around in the lower abdomen rather indicates a psychogenic mechanism.
It is useful to inquire about the patient's activities and the length of her working day. One should ask whether the pain starts when she is bending forward (as while making beds or vacuum cleaning) or after prolonged sitting or prolonged standing; whether the pain awakes her in the morning; whether she feels a rigidity in the lower back when she gets up, what increases the pain, and how she can relieve it; whether she has had to interrupt her usual activities or her professional work. One should also inquire whether she has been receiving any compensation and whether there is any dispute or litigation related to her present condition.

4.2.2 Somatic Examination

A *general physical examination* will be indicated when the cause of the pain is not immediately obvious or when, besides the pain complaint, there are also symptoms, such as fatiguing easily or losing weight. Even when there are indications of a psychogenic condition, a careful general physical examination is necessary as there may be a coincidence of somatic and psychogenic disturbances. Moreover, the physical examination proves to the patient that her complaints are taken seriously and it may constitute a good introduction to a psychological evaluation if this is deemed useful or necessary.
Examination of the abdomen will start with a deep palpation. When the pain localization is rather sharply circumscribed, performance of an elective palpation of the abdominal wall is indicated to find out whether the pain is parietal.
The exploration of low backache calls for a careful orthopedic examination; this is described in detail in Chap. 16.
During the combined abdominovaginal examination, one should look for the most frequent causes of gynecologic pain. Attention should be paid to the following possibilities: sensitivity of the vaginal inlet, prolapse of the vaginal walls or of the uterus, localized sensitivity along the course of the urethra, which may indicate a urethral diverticulum, a painful scar in the vaginal wall, constitutional or acquired shortness of the vagina.
At the level of the cervix and the vaginal vaults, it is important to look for the presence of a chronic cervicitis, from which the inflammatory process may spread into the parametrial tissues, or a cervical scar that has extended in a vaginal vault, or tenderness of the posterior parametrium with or without small rice-grain-like (endometriosis?) or anteroposterior condensations (actual or past posterior parametritis?) in the posterior paracervical cellular tissue. Extreme tenderness of the posterior vaginal vault and extraordinary mobility of the cervix ("universal joint cervix") are said to be characteristic of the Allen and Masters syndrome. We believe this syndrome to be very rare. The position, size, shape, sensitivity, and mobility of the uterus are noted on palpation. If the uterus is retroverted, one should ascertain whether it is mobile or fixed.

It should also be noted whether the adnexa can be palpated, whether they are normal or increased in size, sensitive, mobile, or fixed. Care should be taken not to consider as a painful adnexum a sensitive strand of tissue or a scar in a lateral or posterolateral parametrium; this may lead to an erroneous diagnosis of chronic adnexitis. Furthermore, one should not consider a lowlying cecum or a loop of the sigmoid colon as an enlarged and sensitive adnexum.

4.2.3 Some Special Explorations

Hysterography can be a useful tool in studying the pathogenesis of essential dysmenorrhea (Youssef 1958 a, b). It may be indicated to explore the uterine cavity in secondary dysmenorrhea when a submucous fibroid is suspected, or a congenital malformation of the uterus, or some intrauterine pathology, such as traumatic intrauterine adhesions (Asherman's syndrome) or intrauterine adhesions due to genital tuberculosis. Hysterography – preferably with a water-soluble medium – makes it possible to search for intramyometrial expansions suggestive of adenomyosis.

A hysterosalpingography may sometimes reveal an endosalpingiosis of a tubal stump in a postsalpingectomy painful condition (Palmer 1970) or a hydrosalpinx. It may also show tubal lesions compatible with genital tuberculosis. There is, however, a possibility of reactivating a pelvic inflammatory disease or causing a septic infection of a tubal tuberculosis; consequently, whenever these conditions are suspected, a laparoscopy may be preferable.

In continental Europe, some authors believe that pelvic varicosities are a frequent cause of pelvic pain and therefore perform a phlebography of the pelvic veins by injecting a water-soluble medium transmyometrially or via other routes. We have no personal experience with pelvic phlebography. In Chap. 18, it will be emphasized that one should be very cautious about ascribing chronic pelvic pain to pelvic varicosities.

Furthermore, pelvic varicosities can be detected almost as well by laparoscopy, a far more useful diagnostic tool in cases of chronic pelvic pain.

4.3 Gynecologic Laparoscopy

Although the limits of bimanual examination in exploring the female genitalia had been realized for a long time, they have become even more clear since we have been able to compare the data obtained by bimanual examination on the one hand and by laparoscopy on the other. As borne out by many publications, chronic lower abdominal pain ranks among the most important indications for diagnostic laparoscopy.

Table 2 gives the major indications in a series of some 21 000 diagnostic laparoscopies studied by the R.C.O.G. Enquiry into Gynaecological Laparoscopy (Chamberlain G and Brown J. C, 1978)

It is not our intention to enter into the technical details of laparoscopy and the precautions to be observed. They are explained at length in several excellent books and atlases, e.g., Palmer (1975), Steptoe (1967), Phillips and Keith

Table 2. Diagnostic laparoscopy by major indication (R.C.O.G. Enquiry 1978)

Major indication	No.	%
Infertility	9048	43.1
Pain	10825	51.7
Infertility and pain	186	0.9
Menorrhagia	84	0.4
Ovarian enlargement	389	1.9
Lost IUD or other foreign body	156	0.7
Other	283	1.3
Total	20971	100.0

(1974), Cremers and Hoynck van Papendrecht (1976), Frangenheim (1977), and Semm (1977).

It should be stressed that laparoscopy has to be performed in a systematic way and that it is important to be cautious in the interpretation of the observed data. In the field of chronic pain, there is indeed a frequent gap between visual observation and diagnostic conclusion.

4.3.1 Systematic Visual Exploration of the Pelvis

An efficient visual exploration of the pelvis presupposes that the uterus can be elevated and moved laterally by a hysterography cannula or by a suction intrauterine cannula of Semm. The adnexa can be explored by a palpator or an atraumatic forceps or a suction probe (of Semm); these instruments may be introduced either through the laparoscope or through a small trocar, which is inserted by means of a second puncture.

A drawing of the most important data observed during laparoscopy is as good as, or better than, a meticulous description. An example is provided by Fig. 8, which represents the scheme that has been in use for many years in the Human Reproduction Unit of our Department.

The following is a description of the data that are useful to gather during a laparoscopy. Their importance in the explanation of the pain will be discussed later.

To observe any *pelvic varicosities* in the infundibulopelvic ligaments or along the basis of the broad ligaments, the pneumoperitoneum, the trocar and the laparoscope should be inserted with the patient in the horizontal position; the patient should then be inclined as quickly as possible into a steep Trendelenburg position. When the uterus is elevated, it is easy to observe any varicosities present; it takes at least 1 or 2 min before varicosities will empty themselves.

Adhesions in the pelvis between intra-abdominal and pelvic organs, or at the level of the cecum or the sigmoid colon, should be noted together with their characteristics. Are they wide or thin or threadlike? Are they likely to be lax or tense when the patient is in the upright position? Are they likely to interfere

Name________ Chart No.______

Indication______ LMP__________

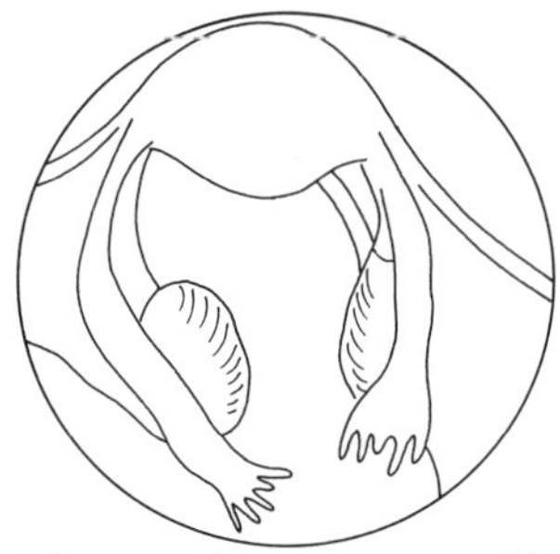

Left Tubes Right

Isthmic part

Ampulla

Methylene blue test

Ovary:

Douglas:

Uterus:

Biopsy:

Aspiration of peritoneal fluid

Photograph

Conclusion

Date of next menstruation________

Gynecologist____________

Fig. 8. Data sheet for laparoscopy

with the function of the organ to which they are attached? If it is felt that the adhesion may contribute to the pain and if it can be sectioned by laparoscopic means, it is of course preferable, both from a diagnostic and from a therapeutic viewpoint, to section it forthwith. In this connection, it is useful to call attention to the dangers of using high-frequency current for this type of work. This is made quite clear by Semm (1977) in a section on "Electricity and Laparoscopy" in his *Atlas of Gynecologic Laparoscopy and Hysteroscopy*. When adhesions cannot be sectioned, it will be useful, at the end of the laparoscopy, to examine their degree of tension when the patient is again in the horizontal position and when most of the gas of the pneumoperitoneum has escaped.

The color, size, and shape of the *uterus* should be observed and the presence of fibroids, if any, should be established. If the uterus is in retroversion, it should be verified whether this is mobile or fixed and, if fixed, whether the cause may be endometriosis, pelvic inflammatory disease (PID), genital tuberculosis, or something else.

The *tubes* should be followed from their uterine end to their lateral end. Any signs of inflammation, nodularities, distension, and adhesions are to be noted. If the peritoneal covering of the tubes looks inflamed or if a tube is enlarged, pressure on the tube with a palpator will sometimes squeeze a drop of pus out of the fimbrial end, indicating an acute or subacute salpingitis. Torsion of the pedicle of a hydatid of Morgagni can be responsible for a severe episode of pain in an iliac fossa; in such a case, there will be a necrotic hydatid at the end of its twisted pedicle. A torsion of a hydatid has sometimes been mistaken for appendicitis.

Attention should be paid to the size, shape, color, and mobility of *the ovaries.* To examine their mobility, they may be lifted up with a palpator or with a suction probe. Probing the mobility is important in the evaluation of an infertility case. It is equally important in pain syndromes, as foci of endometriosis may go unrecognized when the lower surface of the ovary adheres to the posterior leaf of the broad ligament. Endometriosis of the ovaries may take various forms: as blue or black, scar-like implants, as blue-domed or brownish cystic tumors, or as a brown line of demarcation between an adherent ovary and the underlying peritoneum. An ovarian endometriosis may be buried in a magma of adhesions. A chocolate cyst may sometimes be hidden under the rather thick white tunica albuginea of an enlarged ovary. In this case, it will only be recognized if it is adherent to the posterior leaf of the broad ligament; if it is not, an enlarged ovary can be punctured to examine its contents.

Small cysts of the ovary may have a varied origin, which is not always easy to recognize on inspection. It is in fact not easy to distinguish between one or more follicular cysts, a benign or malignant cystic tumor, or an endometriotic cyst. Puncture of the cyst with aspiration of its contents and cytologic examination will frequently be helpful in the differentiation. The cytologic examination should be done as soon as possible to remove without undue delay any malignant tumor discovered by the cytology of its contents. A small tumor that laparoscopy suggests has characteristics of malignancy should, however, not be punctured; instead, a cytologic examination of the peritoneal fluid aspirated from the pouch of Douglas is called for.

Aspirating the *fluid from the pouch of Douglas* for cytologic examination is always useful, as it may reveal signs of inflammation or microscopic signs of endometriosis. When there is a great amount of fluid, it is helpful to empty the pouch of Douglas to make visual exploration easier.

Any endometriotic lesions found in the pelvis should be carefully described. It should be noted whether they extend superficially or are surrounded by a fibrotic capsule and penetrate into the depth of the tissues, whether the lesion is "closed" or open, and whether the endometriosis has given rise to adhesions that disturb the function of the tubes, the ovaries, or segments of the large or small intestine. Indeed, the characteristics of the lesions will indicate whether they are causal factors in the chronic pain syndrome of the patient. In some cases, a small biopsy of a lesion will help to verify its nature, endometriotic or otherwise.

Blood in the pouch of Douglas may have various origins depending on the phase of the menstrual cycle. It may stem from a retrograde menstruation, from a bleeding superficial endometriotic lesion, from a ruptured follicle, or from adhesions torn during the elevation of the uterus. If a thin layer of clotted blood is found on the omentum or on the intestine, it may also come from the puncture wound in the abdominal wall.

Many gynecologists after Allen and Masters (1955) have considered tears or depressions in a uterosacral ligament or in the posterior leaf of a broad ligament

to be causes of chronic lower abdominal pain. As we shall see later, there are several reasons for seriously questioning this causal relationship.
Finally, the laparoscope should also be directed toward the sigmoid and the ascending colon, toward the appendix, and toward the terminal part of the small intestine. Indeed, it may be necessary to evaluate the significance of adhesions, and lesions suggestive of Crohn's disease may be discovered. In recurrent left iliac fossa pain in women over 40, laparoscopy may make it possible to differentiate between a lesion of the left adnexum and a peridiverticulitis. It may also reveal a plausible cause for an intermittent intestinal subocclusion and, though very rarely, may show a torsion of an epiploic appendix of the rectosigmoid.

4.3.2 Indications

Laparoscopy cannot and should not replace a detailed history and a careful clinical examination. Laparoscopy requires general anesthesia and entails certain risks, which are duly stressed in the books on laparoscopy referred to above. Although thousands of laparoscopies are being performed the world over, it should not be forgotten that a patient may die from it. One should therefore be aware of the contraindications, and there should always be a valid indication.
Examples of indications in the study of chronic pain syndromes are:

1) Necessity of differentiating between a gynecologic and nongynecologic cause of chronic and lower abdominal pain
2) Inconclusive results of the clinical examination
3) An unsuccessful treatment trial after a clinical probability diagnosis
4) Slightest doubt of a serious or malignant disorder
5) Need to reassure an anxious patient

4.3.3 Contraindications

Contraindications are related either to the general health of the patient or to local abdominal conditions. They include:

1) Some cases of severe cardiac or circulatory insufficiency, which will make the anesthesiologist object to general anesthesia during which a Trendelenburg position and an increase of the intraperitoneal pressure will be required.
2) Two or more previous median subumbilical laparotomies, especially when extensive adhesions have been found during or are presumed to have developed following earlier explorations.
3) Suspected tuberculous peritonitis.
4) Suspected extensive intra-abdominal carcinoma, in which case an exploratory laparotomy is likely to be less dangerous than a laparoscopy.

When, due to the possibility of adhesions, there is doubt about the safety of the procedure, the precautions suggested by Semm (1977) are to be recommended:

1) Puncture of the abdominal wall with a Verres needle, to which an open syringe half filled with sterile physiologic saline solution has been attached.
2) Injection of 6-8 ml of a sterile saline solution followed by an aspiration test, which should be negative.

4.4 Interpretation of Data: Some Causes of Diagnostic Errors

Diagnostic errors may have various causes. They may be due to carelessness in the examination. Patients have undergone a salpingo-oophorectomy for a supposed pain in the left or right iliac fossa, whereas in fact the pain was localized either in the left or right groin or in the left or right flank. Neglect or insufficient consideration of important biologic data, such as a slight fever, a slight hyperleukocytosis, or an accelerated blood sedimentation rate may be reasons for missing an acute or subacute pelvic inflammatory condition.

Too frequently the first anomaly found during examination is accepted as the cause of the symptom. However, one should always await the results of all the examinations prescribed and consider critically the possible causal relationship between the symptoms and signs on the one hand and the structural or functional anomalies discovered on the other. If, for example a roentgenologic examination of the lumbosacral spine reveals an abnormality in a patient with low backache, this merely raises – but does not solve – the question of whether the anomaly explains the pain. This problem is well-known to orthopedists.

It is useful to recall that combined pains, i. e., pain complaints that are due to two different causes, are not uncommon and that a complete cure will probably not be achieved by taking care of only one of the causal conditions.

In some chronic pelvic pain syndromes, no obvious pathologic anomaly will be found. It is possible in such cases that two or more factors contribute to the pathogenesis and that psychological influences may not be the least. It is therefore imperative to examine the psychosocial background and the current behavior of the patient and not to resort to surgery too easily. A good deterrent against operating too readily is to reexamine, at regular intervals and for at least 2 years after the operation, all the patients with chronic pelvic pain that have undergone surgery.

References

Allen WM, Masters WH (1955) Traumatic laceration of uterine support. Am J Obstet Gynecol 70:500-513

Chamberlain G, Brwon JC (1978) Gynaecological Laparoscopy. Report of the Confidential Enquiry into Gynaecological Laparoscopy. Royal College of Obstetricians and Gynaecologists, London

Creemers HP, Hoynck van Papendrecht HPCM (1976) Laparoskopie in de interne Geneeskunde en Gynaecologie. Stafleu, Leiden (Laparoscopy in internal medicine)

Frangenheim H (1977) Die Laparoskopie in der Gynäkologie, Chirurgie und Pädiatrie. Thieme, Stuttgart

Palmer R (1970) Laparoscopy in diagnosis and treatment of endometriosis and pelvic adhesions. Ned Tijdschr Verloskd 70:293-296

Palmer R, Palmer E (1975) Les explorations fonctionelles gynécologiques, 2nd edn. Masson, Paris

Phillips J, Keith L (1974) Gynaecological laparoscopies. Stratton, New York, London

Semm K (1977) Atlas of gynecologic laparoscopy and hysteroscopy. Saunders, Philadelphia London Toronto

Steptoe PC (1967) Laparoscopy in gynaecology. Livingstone, Edinburgh London

Sternbach RA (1974) Pain patients. Academic Press, New York
Woodforde JM, Merskey H (1972) Personality traits of patients with chronic pain. J Psychosom Res 16:167-172
Youssef AE (1958a) The uterine isthmus and its sphincter mechanism, I. The uterine isthmus under normal conditions. Am J Obstet Gynecol 75:1305-1319
Youssef AE (1958b) The uterine isthmus and its sphincter mechanism, II. The uterine isthmus under abnormal conditions. Am J Obstet Gynecol 75:1320-1332

5 Psychological Aspects of the Pain Experience (P. Nijs)

5.1 General Considerations

Every pain experience has psychological aspects. Regardless of its localization, pain is usually considered as something having to do with damaged tissue; it is thus generally held to have an organic origin, a view shared by many doctors and patients.

And yet it is not self-evident that pain must be due to somatic lesions. Feeling pain is an experience; it is a subjective response to an unpleasant stimulus, which the patient will localize somewhere in her body. However, this stimulus may be somatic or psychological (Buyse 1974), and the doctor must constantly keep in mind that the pain experience is a highly ambiguous clinical datum.

Most patients equate being ill with being somatically ill. All social classes, but especially the lower ones, are reluctant to accept psychological (e. g., neurotic) disturbances as diseases, although it must be conceded that the upper classes are somewhat more tolerant of complaints about psychological problems (e. g., anxiety or depression). However, pain is immediately accepted as a symptom of somatic illness. Consequently, pain will frequently be the complaint of a woman who "wishes" to be considered as ailing, either because of a somatic lesion or because of other problems threatening her well-being, be they psychological, social, professional, familial, or sexual.

Thus far, the mechanisms by which psychogenic factors cause or influence pain complaints have mostly withstood elucidation, a fact that makes many doctors feel ill at ease or even irritated.

In our terminology, the concept of psychogenic gynecologic pain primarily means pain that can be shown to be related to emotional factors, although the nature of this relation may as yet not have been elucidated.

Two broad types of psychogenic pain can be distinguished. A patient may have a bodily reaction to the stress, the psychological tensions under which she lives (e. g., tension headache, colon dysfunction, tension backache), or a patient may try to "solve" a psychological problem by means of a somatic pain complaint. In this way, she converts the psychological problem into a bodily symptom, which thereby acquires meaning; in other words, it becomes a symbol (body language). The pain is made to serve a specific purpose, which finds no verbal outlet. For example, a patient who consciously forgives her husband's infidelity may subse-

quently complain of dyspareunia: pain converted into body language because she no longer desires coitus with her husband and under these circumstances she may no longer have to submit to coitus. This is a "solution" that allows the patient to present somatic complaints and to circumvent the conflictual aspect of the problem. Such behavior may well appear insincere or exaggerated and make the doctor feel that her pain is imaginary, but he must never consider it to be simulated. Simulation, i. e., active and conscious feigning of a nonexistent pain complaint, is rare. Whatever the findings – or lack of findings! – a doctor must never give the impression of not believing in the reality of the pain complaint.
Indeed, to feel pain is to experience it, and no matter what its genesis, for the patient pain is a true experience, against which she is as powerless as any human being against an emotion that overwhelms them. For this reason, a doctor should not only undertake a careful physical examination of a patient with a pain complaint but should equally thoroughly observe her behavior.

5.2 Behavioral Patterns of Patients with Acute and Chronic Pain

Patients with acute pain behave quite differently from patients with chronic pain. A patient with acute pain experiences anxiety, both about the cause and the severity of the pain. Pain is a signal, experienced in the body, of a threat; acute pain means an acute threat, and the severity of the pain indicates the severity of the threat.
The behavior of such a patient therefore follows a pattern of "emergency response": she has a so-called fight or flight reaction, which will subside only when she has been given adequate treatment or a reassuring explanation. Acute pain is accompanied by an increased tone of the striated muscles, by mydriasis, accelerated breathing, palpitation, increased blood pressure, and perhaps transpiration, a dry mouth, etc. It will be immediately obvious to the doctor that such a patient is in pain and is anxious. In fact, even if the patient does not confirm this, the pattern just described is the typical pattern of anxiety. In addition, the pain sensation is diminished by measures tending to reduce anxiety, such as tranquilizers or reassurance.
A patient with chronic pain behaves differently. Pain that drags on for months will change a patient's reaction to it. Patients with acute pain keep, or try to keep, a certain distance vis-à-vis their pain. They feel pain in a particular part of the body, in a particular area, in a precise spot; it is as though the pain is observed externally.
In cases of chronic pain, however, this psychological distance is lost: "the patient is in pain, she is surrounded by it, it absorbs her and dominates everything." The world in which she lives gradually shrinks down to the experience of her own body: her interest in her family or friends, work, or hobbies declines continually. In the center of her preoccupations is the pain and what it involves: visits to the doctor, medical examinations and prescriptions, surgery, confrontation with health insurance company officials, etc. Her entire existence is reduced to the pain experience. This indifference to the world around her and preoccupation with her own body is often accompanied by a number of vegetative symptoms: loss of appetite, sleep disturbances, decreased zest for work and life, irritability,

decreased libido, etc. Taken together, these symptoms are fairly typical of a depressive behavioral pattern. In fact, as will become clear later on in this study, antidepressants can decrease the pain in some cases, just as analgetics can alleviate the depressive reaction.

5.3 Presentation of the Pain Complaint

5.3.1 Verbal Presentation

Verbal behavior is an important constituent of pain behavior; the doctor must therefore pay careful attention to the language the patient uses to describe her pain.

As all behavior comprises learning aspects, pain complaints can vary greatly owing to social and cultural factors. For example, it is well-known that southern European patients will in general behave noticeably more emotionally than central or northern European women who tend to express themselves more reservedly and soberly. Specifically, as for learning how to react to pain, a women who grew up in a family in which the mother and/or elder sisters regularly and ostentatiously suffered abdominal pain will behave differently from one whose environment was of the opinion that physical discomfort was to go unnoticed.

5.3.2 Indications Suggesting Psychogenic Components in Pain Complaints

These factors may not mean much by themselves, but their association is significant of psychogenic pain.

5.3.2.1 General

The first general impression may be that of an exhausted, depressed patient or that of an anxious, tense, irritable one.

5.3.2.2 Description of the Pain

A rather passive patient, who submits to her pain, will give nothing but a vague, even sparing description. A patient absorbed in her complaints, on the other hand, will talk volubly and in superlatives, using baroque imagery tending toward the fanciful, e. g., "something that crawls around down there in the abdomen, a band of fire around the abdomen." Careful and detailed questioning may sometimes bring to light, instead of actual and real pain, "a feeling of heaviness, of tension, of pressure, of bearing down in the lower part of the abdomen," or its seeming opposite, "a feeling of emptiness in the abdomen." While describing all this, the patient may look as if she is carrying most of the world's woes – or she may put on a mysterious, Gioconda-like smile, which will give the doctor a most unpleasant feeling of powerlessness.

Even though it is impossible to determine solely from the patient's description whether she suffers from psychogenic or somatogenic pain (or both), this description can orient the doctor in a certain direction, which calls for further confirmation by clinical investigation.

Somatic pain is described as a perception. For example, a burn causes a pain sensation that is, so to speak, external to the victim. This sensation is rather like a tactile feeling, a perception of the senses. However, throbbing or piercing pains, which the patient experiences and which penetrate deep into the patient (so-called ego-near pains) and overwhelm a patient like an emotion, are rather indicative of psychogenic pain; even though in both instances the description will use words that designate somatic lesions.

5.3.2.3 Localization

The pain localization will sometimes extend beyond the areas typical of somatic gynecologic pain; its boundaries will then be defined not by anatomy, but by the psychic field of the patient's body image. Thus, a women can describe a pain emanating from her abdomen via her left flank to her left breast, which may be hyperesthetic to pressure or palpation.

Sometimes the localization is vague and remains irritatingly so, even after precise questioning, or it may be abnormally accurate, being confined, for example, to one precise point.

5.3.2.4 Concomitant Symptoms

In cases of somatic pain, concomitant symptoms are usually limited. A patient with psychogenic pain, however, is often dysphoric: there is an unpleasant, uncomfortable feeling of tenseness; her attitude, her reactions, and her response to pain will often be vehement or capricious. She may have a long list of complaints, which all fit a diagnosis of depression or exhaustion due to chronic stress (dizziness, nausea, headaches for which the ophthalmologist has prescribed dark glasses). Her neurovegetative instability will be easily noticeable during the examination, revealing itself, for example, in excessive perspiration or in the appearance of red patches on her neck and face. Yet, the pain may be the only symptom so that the doctor will – wrongly – be convinced it is organic.

5.3.2.5 Evolution

The evolution of the pain may be capricious, atypical, and accentuated sometimes by biologic rhythms (e. g., the menstrual cycle), but above all it will be dependent upon the psychic (stress) situation, worsening when there are conflicts with her husband, with her parents or in-laws, in her work, etc. Sometimes the doctor will find that the patient's complaint changes from one consultation to another.

5.3.2.6 Attitude

A patient's attitude toward psychogenic pain is different from her attitude toward somatic pain. In the latter case, she will attempt to carry on as usual in spite of the pain, which she will try to get rid of. However, a patient with psychogenic pain loses her perspective and sense of proportion. She becomes absorbed in all sorts of uncomfortable sensations. It is normal for pain to be alarming as long as no sufficient explanation of its origin is forthcoming and as long as no treatment is being applied. However, psychogenic pain continues to occupy the center of the stage and the patient's logorrheic analyses ("I'm perfectly willing but my pain down there is not") will soon try the doctor's patience.

In this way, the complaints are projected outside, there to serve as a stumbling block between doctor and patient. The doctor will often find that the patient is unwilling to listen or reluctant to react adequately to the explanation of the somatic findings. The patient may demand immediate surgical intervention. Feelings of resentment toward official bodies, such as Medicare, health insurance companies, the National Health Service, are not exceptional.

5.3.2.7 Environment

The attitude of the patient's environment, especially that of husband and/or parents, is important. The environment will be helpful and solicitous of a patient with somatic pain, but when there is a history of psychogenic pain, expecially one that drags on and on, their attitude will unavowedly become irritated or resigned, or it may turn overprotective, especially that of the mother or the husband. All this makes manifest how pain plays its unconscious role in (family) relations. For an adequate observation of pain behavior in the clinic, it is therefore imperative that the nursing staff be able to observe interactions between the patient and the "significant others."

History taking and clinical examination yield data that do not correspond with the clinical characteristics of somatic gynecologic pain syndromes. Moreover, clinical examination will reveal the pain threshold to be variable: drawing attention to the patient's pain will lower it; drawing attention away from the pain will increase it. A patient whose entire attention is fixed on pain is likely to show an increased fear of pain. This heightened attention produces an overall increase of "arousal," which can, through anticipation, increase the pain experience. Thus, the doctor will get the impression that the patient reacts too vehemently to physical examination.

5.3.2.8 History

History taking and the data from the file often confirm that the result of physical treatment will depend on the psychological importance attached to it: an injection will prove more effective than a pill, a surgical intervention more effective than an injection (witness, for example, appendectomy or other surgical interventions), but none will be ultimately effective.

Frequently, the impressive file will mention conflicts with doctors of the health insurance company. Sometimes the doctor may be struck by the lack of understanding or cooperation of the patient, although the therapeutic measures to be taken have been throughly discussed with her.

5.3.2.9 Simulation

If a pain patient often gives the impression she is playing a pain game, this will influence the doctor's attitude toward her. The doctor will feel manipulated by the woman who needs to remain a pain patient. She pretends to detest pills; yet, like an addict, she gets the doctor to prescribe stronger analgetics. She pretends she wants to resume her work as soon as possible; yet, like the professional pain patient she is, she gets the doctor to renew her sickness benefit certificates again and again, or she may thoroughly confuse the doctor by first reacting positively and even enthusiastically to treatment, and then by coming back, disappointed and complaining once again.

The doctor who experiences how all efforts are useless will understand all the better how such a patient holds sway over her environment by her pain behavior. She forces her environment to deal with her as with a sick person who suffers pain, from which apparently no one can relieve her. This woman, who in everyday life may not be able to realize her own wishes and expectations, appears to be quite successful in this respect. This may provoke irritation and even feelings of aggression on the part of the doctor; the more so since her behavior may appear fake, like an alibi serving to avoid a job or a sexual relation with which she can cope no longer. This psychological advantage may seem as important to the patient as any material advantage she might obtain from a compensation neurosis. Finally, a doctor may feel particularly irritated with a pain patient who takes on a passive, dependent, and helpless attitude. Her behavior has gotten her more care and more attention from her environment; in the same way, she will lay a claim on the doctor and demand more of the doctor's attention, care, and time.

5.3.3 Main Psychopathologic Syndromes Inducing or Accompanying Gynecologic Pain Complaints

5.3.3.1 Depression

The use of this term is often confusingly vague; however, the syndrome of depression can be summarized as follows. Depression is an affective disorder characterized by a depressed mood, indifference, loss of drive and zest for life, and often accompanied by feelings of guilt, impotence, and inferiority, leading even to ideas of suicide. Depression also entails psychomotor and motor inhibition. *Psychomotor inhibition* is characterized by loss of memory and concentration and by retardation of thinking (sometimes accompanied by monoideism concerning, for example, incurable disease, or by cancerophobia).

Motor inhibition diminishes the versatility of the facial expression (depressive mask), slows down speech and gait, or may cause the patient to sit or lie almost motionless. Anxiety depression, however, may entail restless agitation or continuous fidgeting.

The somatic symptoms are especially noticeable in cases of *vital depression;* they may include a lowered metabolism, a slower pulse rate, cold limbs, constipation, loss of appetite, sleep, and libido, and sometimes menstrual disturbances. Among all the unpleasant bodily sensations, the functional pain complaints are paramount.

The diagnosis of an overt depressive syndrome usually offers little difficulty, and treatment with antidepressants can be started straightaway.

In cases of masked depression, however, the physical symptoms will be prominent, while the psychic ones remain in the background, hiding as it were behind the (functional) physical complaints, in this case, the pain. Such a patient will first consult a general pracititioner or a gynecologist, not a psychiatrist. This can be misleading since the depressive symptoms will appear "dissolved" into the pain complaints. When she complains of loss of zest for life, lack of appetite, sleeplessness, loss of libido, lack of drive and initiative, etc., she will ascribe all this to her pain, even if careful history taking will in many cases reveal mild depressive symptoms before the pain began.

The most frequent pain complaint in cases of depression is headache; next come, in order of decreasing frequency, pains in the chest, the back, and the abdomen. As has already been stated, chronic pain often leads to depression, and depression often leads to pain complaints. Pain and depression interact.

5.3.3.2 Hypochondriasis

A hypochondriac patient is fascinated by, and even lost in, the experience of a physical (or psychic) disturbance (Ladee 1966). The term hypochondriasis refers primarily to the patient's attitude and behavior vis-à-vis her pain, regardless of whether it has a somatic or a psychological origin. Her behavior is characterized by her physical preoccupation with illness, her phobia of being or becoming ill, and finally her unshakable conviction that she is physically ill, which is completely unamenable to reassuring explanation.

Such a patient's entire sphere of interest has shrunk down to her own body, whose sensations, moreover, are no longer natural or self-evident. All this may be provoked by a frightening event, such as a friend's death from cancer, or by a series of disappointments in the patient's family life or in her profession.

Pilowsky (1969) is right in calling this "abnormal pain behavior": the persistence of the complaint and the absolute certainty of being incurably ill preclude any confidence in the doctor, whose explanations fail to register.

5.3.3.3 Hysteria

The term hysteric conversion symptom is mainly used to denote that there is a demonstrable and meaningful link between a certain symptom and an initial emotionally traumatic experience. This emotional conflict is converted into a

physical symptom (pain), which evokes and expresses this conflict („body language").
Hysteric conversion symptoms tend to occur in so-called hysterical women, whose behavior is faked (theatrical, seductive, manipulative, replete with "typically feminine wiles"), egocentric (as a patient she will claim the status of a special patient and demand that all kinds of exceptions be made for her), and infantile (she will try to appear young, look childishly innocent, or naively dependent on the doctor).
Some patients affect "la belle indifference" but may in this way mask anxiety and uncertainty. They have often played a passive masochistic role in their lives, which may have started with an unhappy marriage and with frigidity.

5.3.3.4 Anxiety

Anxiety syndromes are often accompanied by pain, the pain complaints then being a bodily incarnation of unrest and frustation. The patient is easily frightened, agitated, her symptoms may include palpitations (even extrasystoles), hyperpnea (which may lead to paresthesia of the lips and fingers and even to carpopedal spasm due to hyperventilation), dizziness, trembling, perspiration, and vasomotor reactions affecting the skin. Such a patient will occasionally push the doctor into an excessively reassuring role. Her anxiety can also find its outlet in a single symptom. e. g., cancerophobia.

References

Buyse G (1974) Medizinische Psychologie. Acco, Leuven
Ladee GA (1966) Hypochondrial syndromes. Elsevier, Amsterdam
Nijs P (1969) Psychogene Pijn in de Gynaecologie. Tijdschr Geneeskd 18:897–903 (Psychogenic Pain in Gynaecology).
Pilowsky I (1967) Dimensions of hypochondriasis. Br J Psychiatry 113:84–93
Pilowsky I (1969) Abnormal illness behaviour. Br J Med Psychol 42:347–351

6 Genital Prolapse and Retroversion of the Uterus

6.1 Genital Prolapse

Most patients with genital prolapse have no pain complaints. Some have a sensation of swelling or fullness in the vagina, others feel a dragging discomfort in the lower abdomen. There may be stress incontinence or difficulty in emptying the bladder. These symptoms may or may not be accompanied by low backache; some patients complain of low backache only. In many cases, there is

Table 3. 100 patients with genital prolapse

Degree of prolapse	
Third-degree prolapse	74
Second-degree prolapse	26
Operation performed	
Vaginal hysterectomy	82
Manchester operation	5
Anterior and posterior colporrhaphy	8
Other operations	5
Patients with pain complaints	25

Table 4. Localization of pain in genital prolapse

Dragging discomfort in lower abdomen	7
Pain in lower abdomen and low back	8
Low backache only	10

no correlation between the physical findings and the severity of the patient's complaints.

All these symptoms are relieved by lying down or by reposition of the organs by means of a well-fitting pessary. If the symptoms disappear after insertion of a pessary, the patient will most probably be relieved by operative correction of the prolapse.

With Van de Wiele (1956) we examined the case histories of 100 patients with severe genital prolapse.

Table 3 gives some details of 100 patients with genital prolapse, whose case histories were analyzed from the viewpoint of their pain complaints. Table 4 gives the localization of the pain in the 25 patients with pain complaints.

6.1.2 Pain Mechanisms

The dragging discomfort of the first seven patients was probably due to traction exercised by the prolapsed uterus or bladder on the anterior part of the parametrium (retinaculum uteri). The eight patients with lower abdominal and low back pain should be divided into two groups according to the different localizations of their low back pain. In four of them, the back pain was localized in the sacrogluteal zone and could be explained either by traction on both the anterior and posterior parametrium or, at least in premenopausal patients, by circulatory disturbances favored by the downward displacement of the genital organs.

However, in the four other patients, the backache was lumbar. This lumbar pain may have been of urologic or orthopedic origin. Several authors (Everett and Sturgis 1940; Tandler and Halban quoted in Everett (1947) Gynaecological and obstetrical urology) have shown that in genital prolapse a stricture of the ureter in its course through the basal part of the broad ligament may cause a hyd-

roureteronephrosis. However, this urologic complication probably does not explain the lumbar pain of our four patients; indeed, a slowly progressing dilatation of the renal pelves and ureters is usually a silent process, and pain due to hydroureteronephrosis would not be confined to the lumbar region only, but would also be felt in the flanks and along the course of the ureters.
It is, moreover, interesting to note that in nine of our ten patients who complained only of low backache, the pain was also localized in the lumbar region. Therefore, we felt that the pain had an orthopedic origin and that it would probably not disappear after the operation; the more so as the X-ray films of the lumbosacral spine showed signs of spondylosis and spondylarthrosis in most of these patients. In fact, the lumbar pain had disappeared in eight of the nine patients when they were interviewed several months after the operation. We nevertheless suppose that the lumbar pain was of orthopedic origin and that it was probably due to the influence of the prolapse on the posture and gait of the patients and apparently not directly related to the spondylosis or spondylarthrosis.

6.2 Retroversion and Retroflexion of the Uterus

During the past 100 years, there has been much ebb and flow in the opinions on the pathogenetic role attributed to uterine retroversion. One hundred years ago it was held responsible for a great many diverse symptoms, and uterine suspension was a frequently performed operative procedure. In the beginning of the present century, however, it became gradually clear that most of these operations had little or no effect on the complaints of the patients and there was a strong reaction against overvaluing retroversion, led in Europe by Mayer, Sellheim, and von Jaschke (von Jaschke 1944). At the height of the reaction, some authors even stated that uterine retroversion hardly ever causes symptoms. This seems, however, to be swinging the pendulum too far.
We believe that there are a limited number of mobile retroversions that are responsible for some symptoms; this can be demonstrated by the disappearance of the symptoms after correction of the retroversion. Fixed retroversion is distinct from the mobile variety in that it is not possible to find out which of the symptoms, if any, are due to the fixed retroversion itself and which to the condition that maintains the uterus in its fixed position, for example, endometriosis, sequelae of PID, genital tuberculosis, or adhesions.

6.2.1 Which Symptoms May Be Caused by Mobile Retroversion?

In 1955 we examined the clinical histories of some 350 patients with uterine retroversion who where either followed up as outpatients or admitted for treatment to the Department of Obstetrics and Gynecology of Leuven University. For various reasons, a great many of these case histories could not be used. The symptoms of 100 patients with mobile retroversion were noted, and the influence exerted on these symptoms by correction of the retroversion was studied.

Table 5. Pain symptoms in mobile retroversion (100 patients)

Dysmenorrhea	
1st degree	24
2nd and 3rd	9
Dyspareunia	17
Intermenstrual pain	53

All symptoms that formerly used to be ascribed to mobile retroversion were studied: dysmenorrhea, dyspareunia, intermenstrual pain, menorrhagia, disturbances of the menstrual cycle, leukorrhea, frequency of micturition, etc.
The last four symptoms are outside the scope of this study. Suffice it to say that the correction of a mobile retroversion hardly ever has any influence on these symptoms; their causal factor must therefore in general be found elsewhere.
We will concentrate on the relationship between pain and mobile retroversion. Table 5 gives the frequency of pain symptoms in 100 patients with mobile retroversion.

6.2.1.1 Dysmenorrhea

We will dwell only on the nine cases of severe dysmenorrhea. Four had characteristics of primary dysmenorrhea and, as the retroversion had not been corrected in any of these cases, proof of a causal relationship could not be established; however, it is improbable that retroversion is a causal factor in primary dysmenorrhea.
In two other cases, the dysmenorrhea persisted after correction of the retroversion. In the three last cases, there seemed to be a causal relationship as the dysmenorrhea improved after correction of the retroversion, but it should be noted that in those three instances the dysmenorrhea was merely a menstrual exacerbation of intermenstrual pain and could therefore not be called dysmenorrhea in the strict sense (see Chap. 8). Dysmenorrhea is frequently found in patients with fixed retroversion due to endometriosis or to sequelae of PID, but in such patients the dysmenorrhea is most probably related to the causal condition rather than to the retroversion itself. The above data show that mobile retroversion seldom gives rise to dysmenorrhea.

6.2.1.2 Dyspareunia

Seventeen patients had deep dyspareunia. In 15, the retroversion was the cause of the complaints as the symptoms disappeared after correction of the abnormal position of the uterus. The dyspareunia may in those cases have been due either to pressure exerted on a tender uterine corpus or on a prolapsed ovary. In the two other cases, the dyspareunia persisted after replacement of the uterus; it was due to tender sacrouterine ligaments rather than to the retroversion.

6.2.1.3 Intermenstrual Pain

Of the 53 patients with intermenstrual pain, the complaint was not due to the retroversion in 29; it was a combined pain in 4 and probably due to the retroversion in 20 cases.

1. Pain Not Due to the Retroversion (29 Cases)

In some of these patients, the pain was localized in the lower back and had characteristics of an orthopedic or rheumatologic pain. In others, the pain had characteristics of a gynecologic pain but persisted after reposition of the uterus and insertion of a Smith-Hodge pessary. In such cases, a sensitive posterior parametrium is frequently found and is the likely cause of the pain (Chap. 18).

2. Combined Pain

In four cases, the pain was only partially relieved by correction of the retroversion. The remaining pain component was due in two cases to a spondylarthrosis, in one to a scoliosis at the level of the lumbar vertebrae, and in the fourth to a hyperextension syndrome.

3. Pain Due to Retroversion

In 20 cases, the pain seemed to be due to the retroversion as it disappeared after reposition of the uterus. It is interesting to note the characteristics of pain due to a mobile retroversion.

Localization. In eight cases, the pain was localized only in the lower back, and in eight others in the lower abdomen and lower back. In the four remaining cases, the pain was most severe in the lower back, but there was also a ventral localization. When there is low back pain, it is usually felt at the level of the sacrogluteal zone or less frequently at the level of the lower half of the sacrum. When the pain has a ventral as well as a dorsal localization, it is apparently a projection of a deep-seated pain on the lower abdominal wall and the dorsal part of the pelvis; indeed, the patient will frequently report that palpation of the uterus by the vaginal or the rectal route produces the pain she feels spontaneously.

Other Clinical Characteristics. The pain usually starts after a delivery or a miscarriage. It becomes worse during the premenstrual period and mostly disappears or decreases after the 1st or 2nd day of the period. It also decreases with horizontal rest. On pelvic examination, the retroverted uterus is tender and frequently increased in size and softer than normal. Many gynecologists have observed that the size of a retroverted painful uterus dimines after anterior reposition and that it becomes firmer. It is also important to note that the pain that disappears after correction of the retroversion does so gradually during the 2 days following the reposition.

We are not aware of any evidence indicating a "cystic degeneration of the ovaries" due to a protracted retroversion or retroflexion.

Differential Diagnosis. In our opinion, there are no symptoms or signs that are pathognomonic of a pain-provoking mobile retroversion. The symptoms of a painful retroversion are quite similar to those described by some authors as "pelvic congestion and fibrosis" and by ourselves as "chronic pelvic pain without obvious pathology."

A diagnosis of painful retroversion should be considered if the pain has the above-mentioned clinical characteristics, if the uterus is tender, rather large, and soft on palpation, if there are no signs of endometriosis, and if the posterior parametrium is not particularly tender. Even then, a relationship between the complaints and the retroversion will have to be established by the diagnostic and therapeutic test of replacing the uterus and maintaining the corrected position by inserting a pessary.

Pain Mechanism. Some gynecologists believe that in many cases of "painful retroversion" the complaints are manifestations of a neurotic behavior because some patients feel better after reposition of the uterus even when it is again found retroverted on the occasion of a control examination. This is indeed a fairly common experience. It is quite possible that the symptoms sometimes reveal a neurotic behavior or personality; but at this juncture, two remarks are in order. Every therapeutic endeavor entails a percentage of favorable results that are mere placebo effects. On the other hand, disappearance of a patient's complaints within 2 days of reposition of a uterus that, having been tender and softened, becomes painless and firm, definitely points to a pathophysiologic explanation.

Martius (1953) believed that various factors contributed to the genesis of the pain: (1) traction exercised by means of the sacrouterine ligaments of the retroverted uterus on the sensory nerve endings of the posterior pelvic wall, (2) pressure exercised by the uterine corpus on these nerve endings, and (3) passive congestion in the uterine wall resulting from circulatory disturbances due to the abnormal position of the uterus.

Traction can hardly be a factor because in most cases of retroversion no tension is felt in the sacrouterine ligaments, nor is pressure on the nerve endings of the anterior surface of the sacrum the cause. It is well-known that even voluminous benign tumors developing in the pelvis do not cause pain. Considering that the pain takes several hours to disappear after correction of the retroversion and that after reposition the uterus is frequently observed to have changed in size and consistency, circulatory disturbances may be considered a much more likely causal factor. A painful mobile retroversion therefore seems to be the clearest example of "pelvic congestion."

6.2.2 Treatment of Mobile Retroversion

The great majority of mobile retroversions remains symptomless, and no treatment is needed in these cases. In most of them, it is not even necessary to mention to the patient this "abnormal" position, which is found in 15%–20% of all gynecologic patients.

When there are complaints that might be explained by the retroversion, a "reposition and pessary test" should be performed to examine whether there is a causal relationship. Reposition of the uterus may sometimes be difficult in a nonanesthetized patient; it is then worthwhile to perform an examination under anesthesia together with a laparoscopy to verify whether the retroversion is fixed and to try reposition under anesthesia. If the test is positive, the uterus will frequently remain in the corrected position when the pessary is removed after 4–6 weeks. In other cases, the pain disappears even though the uterus is again found in retroversion. Therefore, an operative correction of a mobile retroversion is only indicated in the rare cases in which the complaints recur together with the retroversion after withdrawal of the supporting pessary. When a suspension operation has to be performed, attention should be drawn to 2 technical details:

1) Instead of pulling the round ligament through the anterior abdominal aponeurosis, it is preferable to pull it through the peritoneum at the level of the internal inguinal ring, lead it between the belly of the rectus muscle and its anterior sheath, and suture it to the inside of the rectus sheath (Mattingly 1977). Pulling the ligament through the anterior abdominal fascia may result in postoperative parietal pain (see Chap. 7).
2) The same technique guarantees that the gap left between the stretched ligament and the lateral part of the peritoneal covering can be as small as possible.

6.2.3 Fixed Retroversion

When a fixed retroversion is accompanied by symptoms, it is usually impossible to prove which ones are due to the retroversion and which are not. Treatment must therefore primarily be directed against the causal disorder, and a suspension operation should only be undertaken when conservative treatment has not helped the patient, when there are other indications for surgical intervention (e.g., tubal surgery for infertility), or when the retroversion itself is probably the cause of the complaints, as in some cases of deep dyspareunia.

References

Everett HS, Sturgis WJ (1940) The effect of some common gynecological disorders upon the urinary tract. Urol Cut Rev 44:638

Jaschke RT von (1944) Die Lageänderungen des weiblichen Genitales. Seitz L, Amreich AI (eds) In: Biologie und Pathologie des Weibes, vol IV, 2. Urban & Schwarzenberg, Berlin, pp 115–143

Martius H (1953) Die Kreuzschmerzen der Frau, 4th edn. Thieme, Stuttgart

Mattingly R (1977) Technique of modified Gilliam suspension of uterus. In: The Linde's operative gynecology, 5th edn. Lippincott, Philadelphia Toronto, pp 490–493

Renaer M (1955) Bijdragen tot de studie van de pijn in de gynaecologische praktijk. III. Beschouwingen over de symptomatologie van de retroversio uteri en in het bijzonder over de pijn bij retroversio uteri. Verh K Acad Geneeskd Belg 17:433–457 (Pain in Gynecologic Practice III. The symptomatology of uterine retroversion and, in particular, pain in uterine retroversion).

Renaer M, van de Wiele RL (1956) Les douleurs dans les prolapsus utéro-vaginaux. Bull Soc R Belg Gynécol Obstet 25:172–179

Tandler J, Halban J quoted in Everett (1947) Gynaecdogical and obstetrical urology

7 Parietal Pain

When confronted with complaints of pain in the abdomen, doctors are mainly interested in the diagnosis and the differential diagnosis of diseases of the abdominal viscera; they hardly think of pain that may arise in the abdominal wall. Indeed, most textbooks of internal medicine scarcely mention abdominal pain of parietal origin; moreover, some authors who have studied mechanisms of visceral pain have stressed that abdominal wall hyperalgesia is a common finding in an area of referred pain, whether induced by deep somatic or by visceral disease. These reasons apparently explain why pain arising in the abdominal wall itself without any underlying visceral disease is but infrequently searched for or diagnosed. Yet, on the face of it, it would appear strange indeed if tissues so abundantly innervated as the skin and the fasciae of the abdominal wall hardly ever gave rise to pain, whereas pain due to the various abdominal viscera is a common event. This does not mean that parietal pain is frequent; it is not, however, as rare as many tend to believe. On the other hand, once its existence has been acknowledged, there is a tendency to overestimate its frequency. It is therefore useful to draw attention to its characteristics and its diagnosis while simultaneously damping overenthusiasm by striving toward a critical view of the subject.

7.1 Possible Causes of Pain Arising in the Abdominal Wall

Abdominal pain of parietal origin may be due to various causes that irritate the spinal nerves of the segments T-7–L-1 (Fig. 9). The pain may be due to factors that influence either the posterior columns and posterior horns of the spinal cord, the posterior roots and the spinal ganglia, or the peripheral nerves (Fig. 10).

7.1.1 Posterior Columns and Posterior Horns

Inflammation, tumoral disease, or compression of a posterior column or horn may give rise to a pain radiation into the abdominal wall; this symptom is mostly a component of a severe neurologic disease and therefore seldom seen by gynecologists.

7.1.2 Posterior Roots and Spinal Ganglia

Irritation of posterior roots or spinal ganglia may provoke either an acute or a chronic pain syndrome. This irritation may result from a tumor of a posterior root or from compression either by a collapsed vertebra or by vertebral spurs in patients with spondylosis. According to Judovitch and Bates (1949) and Bates (1950), scoliosis of the spinal column may also provoke radicular syndromes in one or in several adjacent segments of the trunk.

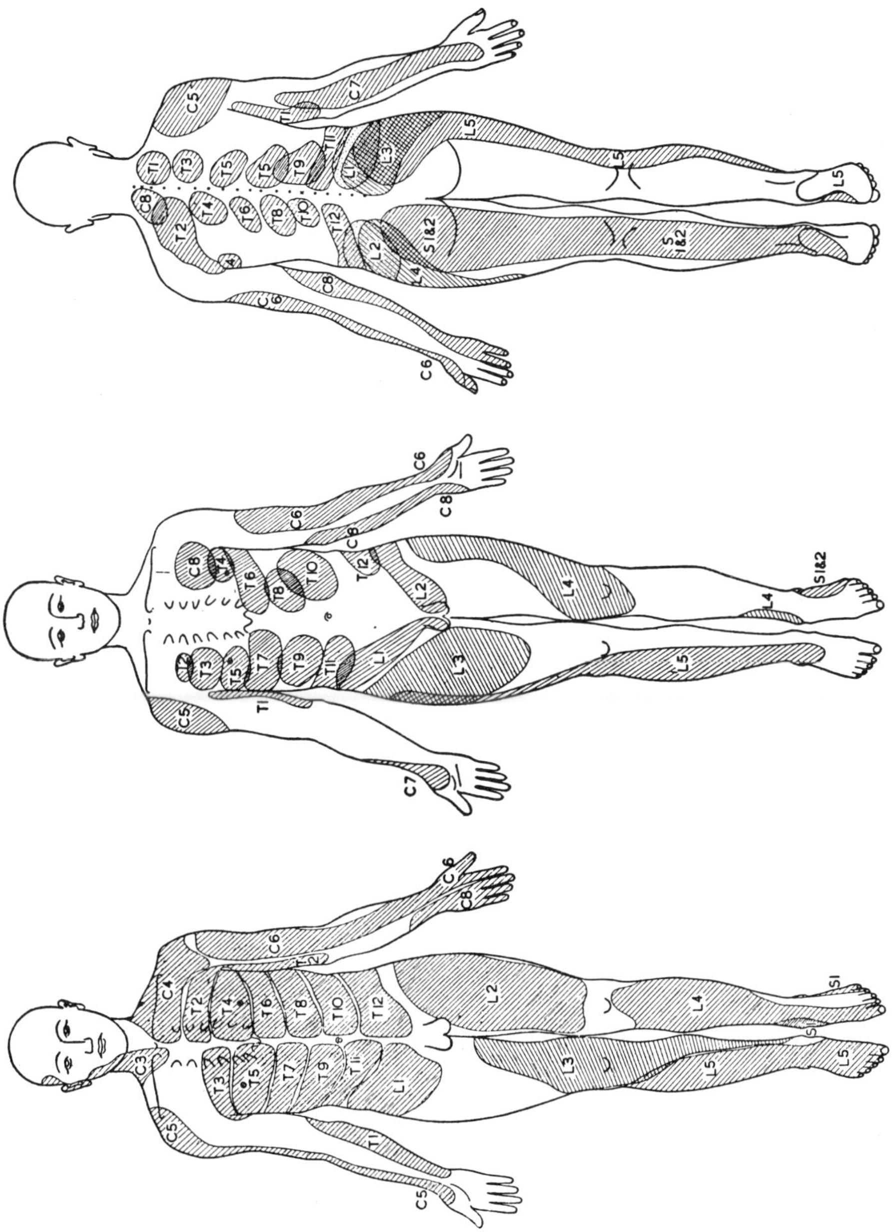

Fig. 9. The two figures to the *right* represent areas of deep pain developed by the injection of the corresponding interspinous ligaments (Kellgren). The *left* figure has been constructed from Foerster's data and represents his "dermatomes." After Th Lewis (1942) Pain. pp 20 and 123. By permission of Macmillan, London and Basingstoke

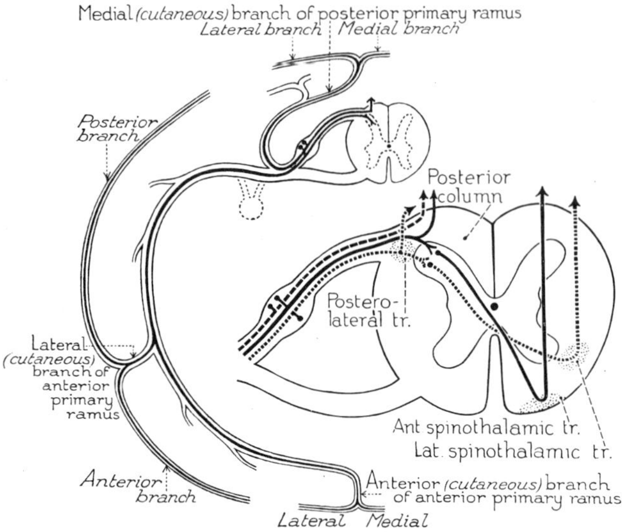

Fig. 10. A segmental nerve, showing the course of sensory neurons from the periphery to the spinal cord. ---- fibers conveying deep sensibility; —— fibers conveying touch; . . . . . fibers conveying pain and thermal sensibility. Haymaker and Woodhall (1956) Peripheral nerve injuries. Saunders, Philadelphia, p 6

Herpes zoster is characterized by a unilateral inflammation of dorsal root ganglia. When herpes zoster occurs between T-7 and L-1, it causes pain in the abdominal wall. It is interesting to mention that it takes 3–7 days for the eruption to appear after the onset of the abdominal pain. In elderly patients, this viral infection may be followed by a severely painful syndrome of postherpetic neuralgia.

In tabes dorsalis, there is selective degeneration in the posterior roots of the spinal nerves and in the posterior columns of the cord; these degenerative changes provoke severe attacks of pain in one or several dermatones. However, tabes dorsalis takes the form of a severe acute pain episode and can hardly be considered a chronic pain syndrome.

Irritation of posterior roots and spinal ganglia has the following characteristics:

- The pain has a radicular distribution, although it is not always felt over the whole area corresponding to the posterior root
- The pain is provoked or increased by mechanical factors, e.g., movements of the spinal column, an increase of the intradural pressure caused by coughing, sneezing, bearing down
- Depending on the causal disease and its clinical course, there may be segmental hyperalgesia, paresthesia, numbness, or hypoesthesia, and finally sensory loss.

7.1.3 Peripheral Nerves

Irritation of the peripheral nerve may be due to pressure, traction, or any other painful stimulus exerted either on the nerve or on the nerve endings.

A diaphragmatic pleuritis, a fracture of one of the lower ribs, or a "slipping rib" can irritate the peripheral nerves and provoke either chronic pain or bouts of acute pain. This pain may be elicited by certain movements or by pressure on a spontaneously tender spot. These factors will only rarely give rise to lower abdominal pain, and gynecologists will therefore hardly ever be confronted with them.

Retroperitoneal inflammations and tumors may also irritate the peripheral nerves of the abdominal wall, but these cases are uncommon. There are also a number of peripheral causes of parietal pain that deserve illustration by a few examples (see Sect. 7.4.2)

7.2. Meaning of Parietal Tenderness in Chronic Abdominal Pain Syndromes

It is well-known that tenderness and muscle guarding of the abdominal wall are found when the parietal peritoneum is irritated during an *acute* inflammatory disease of abdominal organs. In addition, it is assumed that *acute* painful stimuli occurring in an intra-abdominal organ can cause parietal tenderness and contraction of abdominal muscles, even if the parietal peritoneum itself is not directly stimulated; this may be the case in renal and gallbladder colic (Lewis 1942).

Many authors have stated that parietal tenderness is also frequently found in *chronic diseases* of the abdominal viscera. Having carefully examined many patients with chronic pain of gynecologic origin, we feel confident to state that tenderness of the electively palpated abdominal wall is almost never found in these patients. An exception has to be made for those cases in which the parietal peritoneum is also involved in the disease process; in gynecologic practice, this may occur when genital tuberculois has spread to the peritoneum and after rupture of an endometriotic cyst. However, these conditions are rather infrequent.

The parietal tenderness meant here was referred to in Chap. 3. Elective palpation may be performed by two techniques. With Carnett's technique (1926), the patient is asked to contract the abdominal muscles in the manner of bearing down during defecation or during delivery. Another technique, that of Joossens (Renaer and Joossens 1957), is described on pp. 13, 14 (Fig. 7).

A firm pressure exercised on the stretched abdominal wall does not cause pain and, moreover, parietal tenderness as detected by the techniques described above is not found in chronic gynecologic pain syndromes; it may therefore be assumed that parietal tenderness present in a chronic pain syndrome originates in the tissues of the abdominal wall itself.

Although parietal pain is found in only a limited number of patients complaining of abdominal pain, this writer feels that the examination of patients with chronic pelvic pain should routinely include an elective palpation of the abdominal wall to differentiate visceral from parietal tenderness.

If parietal tenderness is found at the site of the spontaneous pain, an anesthetic infiltration of the tender area should be performed, after which an elective palpation will again be done to check whether the pain persists or disappears. If all tenderness has disappeared, the pain is parietal. If the tenderness persists on deep palpation, there is parietal *and* visceral tenderness, which is uncommon.
The coincidence of a visceral pain-provoking cause and a parietal pain at the same site seems to be rare indeed, but it may occur. Therefore, even if parietal tenderness is found, the underlying organ should also be explored for the sake of safety. The coexistence of both pain varieties may be fortuitous. However, as has been shown by the clinical experiments of Jones (1943), there may be reciprocal influence due to convergence and summation of visceral and parietal stimuli at the first synaptic relay area in the dorsal horn of the spinal cord.

7.3 Characteristics of Parietal Pain Due to Irritation of Peripheral Nerves of the Abdominal Wall

- The pain may be continuous with exacerbations; in other cases, it is intermittent.
- Parietal pain localized in the lower part of the abdomen may increase during the premenstrual period. It also increases when sudden pressure is exerted on the tender area, e.g., by the rim of a table or by any other hard object, when the patient stoops or stands up, or when she coughs or sneezes.
- The pain is usually well localized; many a patient will show with one or two fingers the tender area "which could be cut out."

Deep-seated causes, such as a retroperitoneal inflammation or a tumor, may be difficult to diagnose, but they can reveal themselves in general symptoms and signs and, locally, in their repercussions on neighboring organs.
In more peripherally located conditions, the diagnosis can be made when elective palpation of the abdominal wall reproduces the spontaneous pain. The latter disappears after infiltration of the painful site by means of a local anesthetic, preferably together with a depot corticoid. During the infiltration, the pain is exacerbated, but this subsides quickly. The pain may recur for a few hours and disappear thereafter. In other cases, it recurs after a few days or weeks, and a second and even third infiltration may be needed to cure it. In some cases, the pain disappears for the duration of the local anesthesia, but it is not cured by repeated infiltrations. The patient may then be helped either by neurolysis, by section of the nerve tract, or by excision of the pain-provoking focus.

7.4 Some Examples of Parietal Pain in Gynecologic Practice

7.4.1 Pain Due to Irritation of the Posterior Roots and Ganglia

In their book *Analysis of Pain Symptoms as an Aid to Diagnosis,* Janzen and Puff (1966) state: "When thoracic or abdominal pain with a limited extension is not explained by careful exploration of all possible visceral causes, the question arises whether one is not dealing with a so-called segmental neuralgia and a search for a parietal explanation of the pain will be in order."

This author has seen only one example of pain due to irritation of a posterior root. Several years ago, a patient was admitted to the Department of Medicine of the University Hospital with a complaint of pain in her left flank. A cystic tumor was palpated in the left iliac fossa and therefore the opinion of a gynecologist was asked. There was indeed a left ovarian cyst, but it was not tender on palpation and the localization of the pain seemed rather high. Although a left oophorectomy had to be performed, it was felt that the pain could not be explained by the presence of the cyst. Further exploration by the physicians did not reveal another cause for the pain, and a neurologic opinion was sought. In view of the paucity of signs, the neurologist performed a myelography, which showed an intradural tumor. At operation, a neurinoma of the tenth posterior thoracic root was removed.

Judovitch and Bates (1949) have described cases of parietal pain in which the irritation of the posterior root is ascribed either to a scoliosis of the spine or to a disk degeneration. We have been looking for such cases, but have not found any in which the cause was a scoliosis. Of course, it is probable that patients with a severe scoliosis consult an orthopedic surgeon rather than a gynecologist. My orthopedic colleagues tell me, however, that they do not see pain radiations into the abdominal wall in their cases of scoliosis.

The lower part of the abdomen corresponds to the segments and the posterior roots T-10–L-1. As a disk degeneration is rather infrequent at that level of the spine, it is clear that parietal pain in the lower abdomen will only rarely be explained by a degenerated disk. This condition is most frequent at the level of L4–5 and L-5–S-1, but these lesions mainly give rise to low back pain on the one hand and to radiation into the lateral or posterior part of the lower limb on the other. However, we have seen two or three cases in which the patient complained of low back pain radiating not only into a lower limb but also into one or both iliac fossae or into the groin. One of these cases (51 years old) had been complaining for several years of low back pain, which occurred especially when she performed heavy household duties. The pain radiated toward both iliac fossae and into the posterior part of the thighs. Her history revealed several episodes of lumbago. A roentgenologic examination showed a severe degeneration of the L-5–S-1 disk. The gynecologic examination was negative. The low

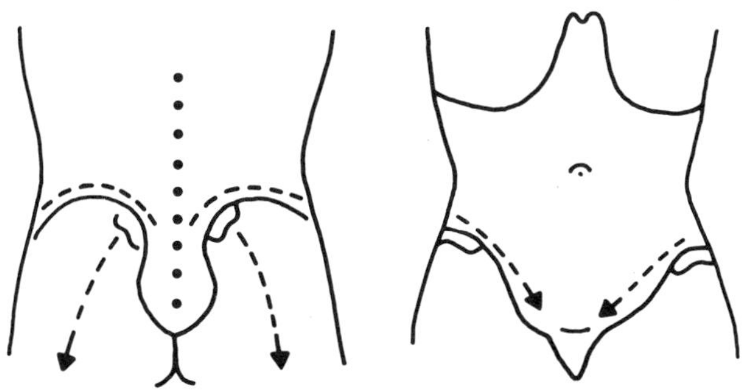

Fig. 11. Dorsal pain localization and abdominal and dorsal radiation in spondylosis (L-5–S-1). Renaer (1971) Chronische pijn in de gynaecologische praktijk. Stafleu, Leiden

back pain and the pain radiating into the lower abdomen and into the posterior part of the thighs improved markedly when she began to wear an orthopedic corset (Fig. 11).

Such cases are interesting from a theoretical point of view. The posterior radicular pain is rather easy to explain, but the pain radiating into the iliac fossae has puzzled us for a long time. Indeed, this pain is not radicular, as it radiates into the area of dermatone L-1, whereas the irritated nerve root is the first sacral. De Sèze (personal communication) has suggested the following explanation: the low back pain is due to stretching of the posterior spinous ligament by the degenerated disk; more laterally, this same degenerated disk irritates the nerve root, which results in pain radiation into the lower limb. The pain in both iliac fossae or in the groin can be explained by pressure of the disk on the lateral rims of the anterior longitudinal ligament. This pain is erroneously localized by the patient in the iliac fossae or in the groin because the sacral promontory lies – like a real promontory – roughly in the center of a transverse section through the lower abdomen at the level of the L-5–S-1 disk.

7.4.2 Pain Due to Irritation of Peripheral Nerves

Parietal pain due to *operative scars* is, of course, well-known. Scars that are most likely to predispose to parietal pain are those after an appendectomy, a Pfannenstiehl incision, a nephrectomy, or a herniotomy. The pain is mostly due to lesions of or adhesions around the ilioinguinal nerve and, less frequently, around the iliohypogastric or the genitocrural nerve. The diagnosis is based on exquisite tenderness on palpation of the scar or of a tender spot in the immediate neighborhood. Meticulous examination may reveal an increased or decreased sensitivity of the skin to noxious stimulation. If infiltration of the painful site with a local anesthetic together with a depot corticoid does not help, the scar may be excised; sometimes a neuroma will be found (Kaeser and von Hochstätter 1973; Staal 1970).

Painful scars due to endometriotic lesions are mentioned in Chap. 11. They are usually particularly painful before and during menstruation, unless the pressure exerted on the tissues is reduced by fistulization of the lesion.

A uterine suspension operation may cause parietal pain when a variant of the Doleris or Gilliams technique is used, in which a loop of the round ligament is pulled through the anterior rectus sheath. In continental Europe, many gynecologists still pull the round ligament through the rectus fascia. We saw at least a dozen patients who complained of pain in the lower abdomen ever since they had undergone a suspension operation. The pain was sharply localized at the site were the round ligaments had been pulled through the fascia. It could be reproduced by elective palpation of the abdominal wall, and the loops of the ligaments could be felt. Several patients were cured by infiltrations of the painful spots with a local anesthetic. In one patient, the suspension operation had relieved her sacral backache, but she had been complaining of two small painful areas in the lower abdomen since her operation. Several anesthetic infiltrations did not cure her pain; finally, we had to excise the loops of the ligaments to relieve it. This sort of iatrogenic pain will be avoided if the loops of the ligaments are brought out around the lateral edge of the muscles and sutured to the innersurface of the rectus sheath.

In elderly people and in patients who are receiving corticosteroid treatment, we should be mindful of *hematomas of the abdominal wall.*

A patient, 60 years of age, came to the outpatient clinic complaning of weight loss and pain in the left iliac fossa. A paramedian tumor of approximately 15 × 8 cm was felt in the lower abdomen, and a carcinoma of the sigmoid was suspected. A barium enema was negative, however. On reexamination, elective palpation revealed that the abdominal wall was not particularly tender, but the tumor seemed to be adherent to the abdominal wall. At laparoscopy, the genital organs were normal, but looking at the undersurface of the anterior abdominal wall, a bluish tumor was found bulging under the parietal peritoneum. Surgical exploration revealed a hematoma due to rupture of the left inferior epigastric vein (Fig. 12).

Kaeser and von Hochstätter (1973) believe that pain along the peripheral part of the ilioinguinal or the iliohypogastric nerve may result from *entrapment neuropathy* due to pressure or traction on the nerve at sites where these nerves perforate the muscles of the abdominal wall. Staal (1970) is somewhat sceptical about functional entrapment neuropathies along the course of these nerves. We are not aware of having met such a functional syndrome in gynecologic practice.

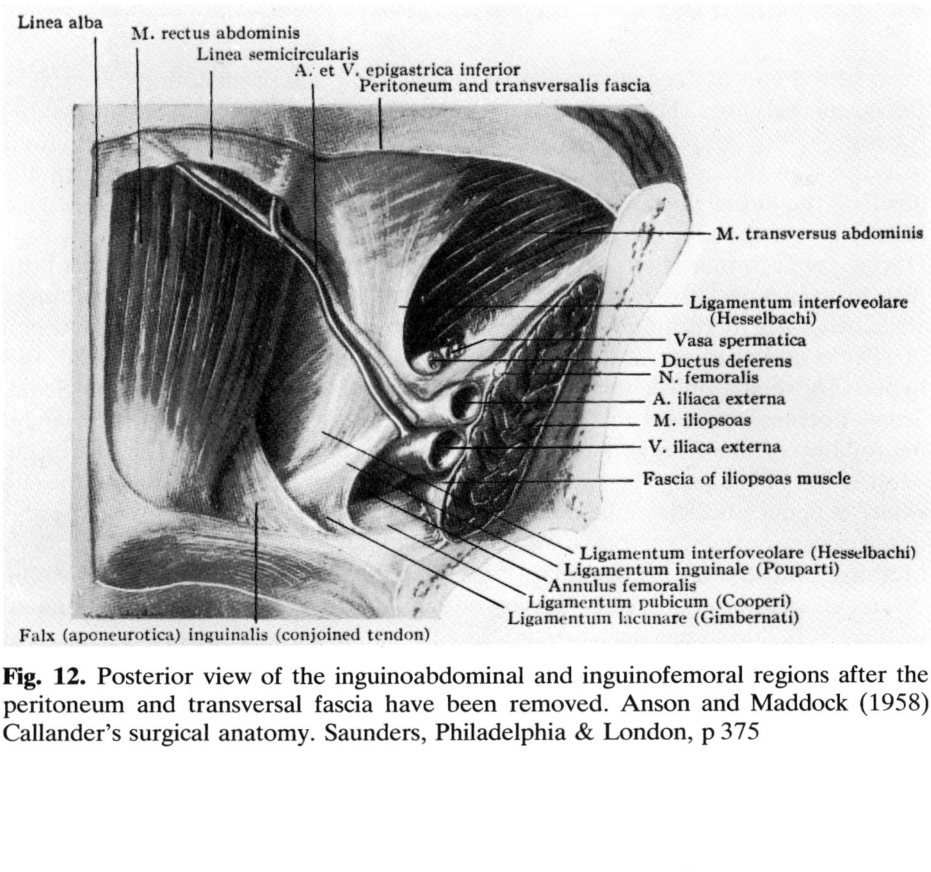

Fig. 12. Posterior view of the inguinoabdominal and inguinofemoral regions after the peritoneum and transversal fascia have been removed. Anson and Maddock (1958) Callander's surgical anatomy. Saunders, Philadelphia & London, p 375

Finally, we have seen about 20 cases in which *parietal pain* was found *without any trace of a scar;* most of them were cured by an anesthetic infiltration, but the pathogenesis of the pain is unclear.

Among these cases, we saw several patients with pain localized about 2 cm lateral to the umbilicus. We almost never found a visceral explanation for this pain, and we cured nearly all by an anesthetic infiltration.

In a few cases, parietal pain was found in the left or right iliac fossa, for example, in a 20-year-old woman who had been complaining for 1.5 years of a gnawing pain at a sharply localized site in the left iliac fossa. Her general practitioner had diagnosed an oophoritis. A gynecologist had found an inflamed cervical erosion and an painful posterior parametrium. Treatment with antibiotics and later electrocoagulation had no effect. Our own gynecologic examination was normal. There was only a slightly painful left posterior parametrium. Elective palpation of the abdominal wall reproduced the pain. Infiltration of the fascia and the muscles at the painful site with 20 ml of a 1% solution of tetracaine (Pontocaine), was performed. During the next 2 days, she had an uncomfortable feeling in the left iliac fossa, after which the pain she had felt for more than 1 year never reappeared.

Parietal pain not related to an abdominaal scar is uncommon, but it has been observed by others (Roberts 1972; Mehta and Ranger 1971) as well as by ourselves. It is perhaps a form of entrapment neuropathy of the terminal perforating branches of nerves of the abdominal wall (Diamond 1977).

7.5 Some Examples of Abdominal Parietal Pain in Obstetric Practice

Toward the end of pregnancy, many patients complain of pain along the rim of the costal cartilages. This pain may be caused by two different mechanisms: (1) traction of the muscles of the distended abdominal wall by their tendinous insertions on the costal grid and (2) pressure exerted on the costal rim by the head of the fetus in cases of breech presentation. This sort of pain can be relieved immediately if it is possible to perform an external version.

During the second half of pregnancy, some patients have cramps in one or both iliac fossae, especially at night. These painful cramps seem to appear at night when the patient turns herself in bed. They have been ascribed by Bushnell (1949) to an irritation of the posterior roots at the level of L-1. However, this hypothesis seems unlikely, as a degenerated disk is uncommon at that level. These nocturnal cramps in the abdominal wall may be due to an entrapment neuropathy of the ilioinguinal nerve. This nerve may be stretched by a brusque contraction of the transverse and the oblique muscles of the abdomen at the site where it penetrates through these muscles. We tell the patient to wear a pregnancy corset at night or to use a close-fitting binder.

Meralgia paresthetica of the superior lateral part of the thigh is another example of an entrapment neuropathy. It may be seen in obese patients and in pregnant women; it is due to pressure on, or stretching of, the lateral cutaneous nerve of the thigh where it passes just anterior to the anterior superior iliac spine.

During the last months of pregnancy, some patients complain of pain localized above the pubic bones and over the pubic symphysis. This pain is due to a relaxation of the pubic symphysis and is part of the "pelvic osteoarthropathy of pregnancy."

Finally, at the subcutaneous ring of the inguinal canal, pain may be provoked during the second half of pregnancy by a swelling, mostly due to varices, which develops around the distal insertion of the round ligament. The swelling and the pain disappear shortly after delivery.

References

Bates W (1950) Abdominal parietal neuralgia. In: Bockus HL (ed) Postgraduate gastroenterology. Saunders, Philadelphia London, pp 256–258

Bushnell LF (1949) The postural pains of pregnancy. West J Surg Obstet Gynecd 57:123–127

Carnett JB (1926) Intercostal neuralgia as a cause of abdominal pain and tenderness. Surg Gynecol Obstet 42:625–632

Diamond AW (1977) Letter to the editor. Lancet II:195

Janzen R, Puff KH (1966) Schmerzanalyse als Wegweiser zur Diagnose. Janzen R (ed) Thieme, Stuttgart, pp 44–54

Jones CM (1943) Pain from the digestive tract. In: Wolff HG (ed) Pain Williams & Wilkins, Baltimore (Proceedings of the Association for Research in Neuroses and Mental Disease, vol XXIII, pp 274–288)

Judovitch B, Bates W (1949) Pain syndromes. Davis, Philadelphia

Kaeser HE, von Hochstätter A (1973) Neurologische Schmerzursachen. Gynaekologe 6:138–144

Lewis (1942) Pain. Macmillan, New York.

Mehta M, Ranger I (1971) Persistent abdominal pain. Treatment by nerve block. Anaesthesia 26:330–333

Renaer M, Joossens JV (1957) Therapeutische en praktische beschouwingen over parietale pijn. Verh Akad Geneeskd Belg 19:55–73 (Therapeutic and practical thoughts on parietal pain).

Roberts HJ (1972) Curable chronic abdominal wall pain. J Fla Med Assoc 59:30–33

Staal A (1970) The entrapment neuropathies. In: Vinken PJ, Bruyn GW (eds) Handbook of neurology, vol VII. North-Holland, Amsterdam, pp 285–325

8 Dysmenorrhea

The term dysmenorrhea refers to painful menstruation. Whereas in many papers on dysmenorrhea quite dissimilar conditions are lumped together, we propose to use the terms dysmenorrhea or algomenorrhea to refer only to episodes of pelvic pain whose duration is limited to the period of menstrual loss or which start 1, or at the earliest, 2 days before and stop 1, or at the latest, 2 days after the blood loss. Pain episodes that start earlier or last longer generally have another pathogenesis and should not be called dysmenorrhea.

8.1 Incidence

The reported incidence varies between wide limits, depending on the definition adopted, the severity of the pain experience, and on the age and socioethnic background of the population studied. It is estimated that between 5% and 10% of all girls in their late teens and early 20s suffer from severe dysmenorrhea during the first hours of their periods (McArthur 1957; Svennerud 1959). Most of them have primary or idiopathic dysmenorrhea; after the age of 25–30, fewer cases of primary and more of secondary dysmenorrhea are found. Dysmenorrhea is the largest cause of absence from work or play in the United States (Sloan 1972).

8.2 Classification

The severity of the pain is variously classified, on a rather subjective basis, as mild, moderate, and severe; by others as mild, severe, and incapacitating; still others distinguish three degrees, where the third degree compels the patient to stay in bed.

From the pathogenetic point of view, it is important to distinguish between primary (essential or idiopathic) and secondary dysmenorrhea. If the pain has a symmetric localization and if no structural anomaly is found on clinical examination, the dysmenorrhea is termed primary, while cases with structural or organic anomalies are classified as secondary.

8.3 Primary Dysmenorrhea

This kind generally begins a few months after menarche; it occurs rarely at the first menstrual period. The gynecologic examination is perfectly normal.

8.3.1 Clinical Characteristics

It is useful, both from the point of view of differential diagnosis and of pathogenesis, to describe the characteristics of the pain. In most cases, the pain starts a few hours or half a day before the beginning of the blood loss. The pain is generally colicky, with cramps every 2–3 min. It is localized either over the whole width of the lower abdomen or in the hypogastrium only; it may radiate toward the sacrogluteal zone. Not infrequently it spreads into the anterior surface of the thighs, but never below the knees. A unilateral localization is quite unusual. During the first few hours of menstruation, there is only slight blood loss, whereas the pain is severe; with increasing blood loss the pain tends to diminish. In a few cases, there are severe cramplike pains during 1 or 2 days before the beginning of the period. In about one-fourth of all cases, the pain is not colicky but continuous and the blood loss rather abundant from the beginning of menstruation. When the pain of primary dysmenorrhea is very pronounced, there may also be nausea, vomiting, and diarrhea.

Dysmenorrhea is assumed to be of the primary variety when the patient is an adolescent, when the pain has the above-mentioned characteristics, and when the gynecologic examination is or appears to be negative. It is, however, worth emphasizing that this assumption will prove to be incorrect in approximately 10%–15% of the cases (Gautier 1976; Parsons and Sommers 1978). Indeed, endometriosis in adolescence is not as rare as used to be thought and may mimic primary dysmenorrhea for months or years.
The rather small size of the uterus of these young patients, some of whom are still virgins, is believed by many doctors and even by some gynecologists to be indicative of uterine hypoplasia or infantilism. However, it is necessary to remember that during the first years after menarche and before the first pregnancy the uterus may be rather small and that its size increases gradually. Hypoplasia and infantilism of the uterus are well-defined and uncommon conditions that should not be diagnosed unless clearly proved.
If no pregnancy occurs, the severity of primary dysmenorrhea tends to diminish after a variable number of years in some patients, but not in all. It disappears in about 80% after the first delivery.

8.3.2 Pathophysiology

To make sure that every case included in a scientific investigation is indeed one of primary dysmenorrhea, it would be necessary to do a laparoscopy on every patient. This is hardly feasible in actual practice, but it should not be forgotten that up to 10% of the cases collected in a clinical series may not be examples of the primary variety. Furthermore, it may be presumed from differences in the characteristics of the pain and from certain therapeutic results (see below) that there is more than one form of primary dysmenorrhea. Therefore it would seem preferable to this writer to group together cases with the same clinical characteristics and to study these. The fact that until now cases with dissimilar clinical characteristics have been lumped together may explain some divergent pathophysiologic observations.

8.3.2.1 Cervical Isthmus

Wilson and Kurzrock (1938) and later Sturgis and Albright (1940) have shown that primary dysmenorrhea is found only at the end of an ovulatory cycle. When a cycle is anovulatory or when ovulation is artificially inhibited, e.g., by an adequate dose of estrogens administered during the first 20 days of a cycle, there will be no dysmenorrhea unless the dose is insufficient to prevent ovulation.
On cervicohysterographies done during the proliferative phase of an ovulatory cycle, the uterine isthmus is relatively wide, whereas it is threadlike and sometimes invisible when the cervicohysterography is performed during the luteal phase. The relative hypotony of the isthmus during the preovulatory phase is in all likelihood due exclusively to the influence of estrogens and its narrowness during the secretory phase to the combined influence of estrogens and proges-

trogens (Asplund 1952; Borell and Fernström 1953; Palmer and Palmer 1963). Hormonal influences also explain why the uterine isthmus is distinctly wider during the second half of an anovulatory cycle and a few days before an episode of dysfunctional bleeding (metropathia hemorrhagica) (Youssef 1958a, b).

Liesse (1947), working with Palmer in Paris, made use of CO_2 insufflations to study the tone of the uterine isthmus in normal women and in patients with primary dysmenorrhea. In three patients with dysmenorrhea examined during a menstrual pain episode, the isthmic tone was distinctly higher than the tone found during menstruation in normal women, indicating that in the patients examined there was a functional hindrance of the menstrual flow. Youssef (1958a, b) confirmed these observations in two very important papers. By injecting 2–3 ml of iodized oil (Lipiodol) directly into the uterine cavity through the posterior vaginal cul-de-sac to perform a "direct" hysterography, he showed that in normal women the tone of the isthmus was highest during the secretory phase and lowest during the proliferative phase.

During the secretory phase the injected Lipiodol passes through the tubes into the peritoneal cavity and does not pass through the isthmus sphincter. In the immediate premenstrual phase, the uterus evacuates itself entirely through the isthmus and the cervix into the vagina and no lipiodol passes through the tubes. In 8 cases with primary dysmenorrhea investigated by "direct hysterography, " no difference from the normal was found during either the follicular or the luteal phase. When the examination took place one or two days before the period, however, it was found that, shortly after the Lipiodol was injected into the uterine cavity, the patient started to complain of severe colicky pains. The uterus did not empty itself as rapidly as it normally does at that particular time and some Lipiodol remained inside the uterus two or three hours after injection; but finally it passed, as it did in normal cases, through the isthmus and cervix and not through the tubes. The isthmus appeared, however, much less relaxed than it was in normal cases in the immediate premenstrual phase.

Youssef therefore concludes that the basic abnormality in primary dysmenorrhea is failure of normal relaxation of the isthmus in the immediate premenstrual period and at the beginning of menstruation.

Confirmation of the above-mentioned observations is found in the work of Mann (1963) who examined, by means of two-stage intrauterine balloons, the relative tone of the uterine corpus and isthmus during the proliferative, secretory, and menstrual phases of the cycle.

The most frequently observed dysmenorrheic mechanism (70% of the cases) was adaptive failure of the isthmus to lose tone at the time of menstruation ... Less frequently observed (10%) but often persisting throughout menstruation was a dysmenorrheic mechanism characterized by myometrial hypercontractility. In such instances, the fundus, in the face of a relaxed isthmic segment, is overly tonic and overly contractile.

Concerning the isthmic factor in the pathogenesis of dysmenorrhea, it is interesting to mention some clinical observations of Polyshuk and Sharf (1965). They examined 35 patients on the 1st or 2nd day of their period by means of culdoscopy. Fifteen patients (group 1) complained of nausea, vomiting, and abdominal pain, which began 24–48 h before the onset of menstraution; eight patients had signs of peritoneal irritation. Twelve patients (group 2) complained of severe abdominal pain, usually cramplike in nature, which began after the onset of the menstrual flow; in one of these patients, the pain was accompanied by nausea and vomiting. Eight patients had no dysmenorrhea (group 3). In the fifteen patients of group 1 and in two of group 2, they found 20–100 ml of blood in the pouch of Douglas. They did not find blood in any of the eight control cases. These observations clearly seemed to be related to isthmic hypertonus.

8.3.2.2 Characteristics of Uterine Contractions

Moir (1934) found that myometrial contractions were stronger during menstruation in dysmenorrheic than in normal women, and although he found signs of relative myometrial ischemia at 120 mmHg, dysmenorrheic pains were felt only when the pressure exceeded 150 mmHg.

Lackner et al. (1937), Wilson and Kurzrock (1938), Liesse (1947), and Diehl and Hundley (1948) found that during menstruation the strength of myometrial contractions and the height of the intrauterine pressure was about the same in normal women and in patients with primary dysmenorrhea. Woodbury et al. (1947) found that intrauterine pressures of 40–80 mmHg associated with dysrhythmic contractions could cause dysmenorrhea, but when contractions were rhythmic, pains were not felt until the intrauterine pressure reached 140–180 mmHg. It should be pointed out that several of the investigations just quoted were performed with small intrauterine balloons, which might well influence the spontaneous contractions of the uterus.

The best measurements of the various parameters of uterine contractions are obtained with the open-tip catheter method developed by Hendricks (1964). With this improved technique, uterine contractions have been studied during the various phases of the cycle in normal women (Moawad and Bengtsson 1967, 1968; Cibils 1967; Hein et al. 1973) and in women with primary dysmenorrhea (Filler and Hall 1970; Åckerlund et al. 1976; Lundström et al. 1976a, b; Csapo et al. 1977; Lundström and Green 1978; Åckerlund 1979). The uterine contractions observed during dysmenorrheic episodes showed various patterns: in some patients, well-coordinated contractions were found with extremely high intrauterine pressures; in other cases "dysrhythmic contractions" with high or low pressures; and in many others the most striking quality was an elevated basal tone between contractions.

Moir (1934) considered his traces to indicate that the pain of dysmenorrhea was due to myometrial ischemia. Åckerlund et al. (1976) recorded, on the 1st day of the period, intrauterine pressures by means of a microtransducer catheter and local uterine blood flow by measuring the thermodilution from a heated thermistor to the blood flow in the surrounding tissues. The continuous component of the dysmenorrheic pain was most pronounced when the myometrial activity showed a comparatively high mean basal tone and when there were only short periods of relaxation between the contractions. The colicky component seemed to occur in association with uterine contractions of high amplitude and accompanying decreases in blood flow. One of their patients reported colicky pain not at times of maximum intrauterine pressure but when there was minimal blood flow.

8.3.2.3 Prostaglandins in Menstrual Endometrium

In the mid 1960s, Pickless et al. (1965) and Pickless (1967) wondered whether primary dysmenorrhea could not be due to the stimulant effect on uterine contractions of the prostaglandins (Pg) F_{2a} and E_2 found in the premenstrual and menstrual endometrium after an ovulatory cycle. Since then, many studies have been devoted to this subject, and several recent reviews have appeared (Halbert et al. 1976; Lundström et al. 1976a, b; Ylikorkala and Dawood 1978). It has been clearly shown, by various methods of measurement, that the prostaglandin content of human endometrium is significantly higher during the luteal than during the proliferative phase (Ylikorkala and Dawood, Table I, p. 839). Lundström and Green (1978) found a mean value of 434 pg $PgF_{2a/mg}$ wet weight (range 192–770 pg/mg) on the 1st day of menstruation in four normal women, but in five dysmenorrheic subjects, the mean was 1625 pg PgF_{2a}/mg (range 270–2664 pg/mg) wet weight of endometrial tissue ($P < 0.05$). On the other hand, no statistical difference was found between the premenstrual levels in the two groups. It has been supposed by several workers that the nausea, vomiting, and diarrhea that frequently accompany severe dysmenorrhea are also due to prostaglandins. Lundström and Green believe, however, that the plasma levels of the prostaglandin metabolites are not high enough to explain these side effects and that high local levels of prostaglandins in the intestinal wall may perhaps be responsible. Much work remains to be done to elucidate the function of various prostaglandins in the pathogenesis of dysmenorrhea (Pickless 1979; Åckerlund 1979).

8.3.3 Pathogenesis of Primary Dysmenorrhea

There has been no dearth of theories trying to explain primary dysmenorrhea. Over the years, most of them have led to different treatment modalities; the search for pathogenetic mechanisms therefore entails more than an academic exercise. Some older theories will merely be mentioned and a few recent ones will be considered more in detail.

The theory of *uterine hypoplasia* as a cause of essential dysmenorrhea has definitively been laid to rest (Jeffcoate and Lerer 1945). The *obstructive theory,* defended by Sims (1866 cited by Davis 1938) under the dictum *"nulla dysmenorrhea nisi obstructiva,"* claimed a structural cervical stenosis hindering the passage of menstrual blood. As such, it has been disproved for a long time but has resurged in the form of functional isthmic hypertony. In the meantime, it caused a great number of operations intending to dilate the cervix and frequently resulting in a more or less severe tear of the uterine isthmus.

According to the *neurogenic theory,* primary dysmenorrhea is due to a neuritis of the superior hypogastric plexus. It was especially advocated by Cotte and Dechaume (1931) and Davis (1938). In Cotte and Dechaume's work and in that of Davis, there were, however, no control obervations on hypogastric plexuses from women without dysmenorrhea, and Skajaa (1951) did not find in the plexuses the examined the neuritic lesions described by Dechaume.

Some authors (Mocquout and Musset 1949) have drawn attention to a local hypersensitivity of the cervix of the uterine isthmus, which can be observed when the cervix is clamped with a tenaculum or when a probe or a Novak curette is introduced through the isthmus. This writer, however, has not been able to convince himself of this kind of *local hypersensitivity.*

An increased pain sensitivity was assumed by Haman (1944) when he felt he had found a lowered pain threshold in dysmenorrheic women. This could, however, not be verified by Javert (1953, personal communication) or by Renaer et al. (1959, unpublished work), who investigated the pain threshold in women with and without primary dysmenorrhea by means of the algesiometer of Hardy and Wolff.

8.3.3.1 Primary Dysmenorrhea – A Psychosomatic Condition?

A failure to find definite pathophysiologic anomalies in former times and ignorance of their existence in recent years has led many authors and numerous doctors to believe that primary dysmenorrhea is essentially a psychogenic condition (Hauser 1960; Lukas 1965; Roemer 1969). We cannot agree with this view: this theory is apparently another example of a psychogenic explanation based on disputable evidence (Lennane and Lennane 1973).

Coppen and Kessel (1963) administered psychometric tests to 500 British women who were in their reproductive period; 12% of these women had severe and 45% had moderate to severe dysmenorrhea. The authors, however, made no distinction between primary and secondary dysmenorrhea. In their conclusion, they stated that

> ...dysmenorrhea is not correlated with neuroticism or extraversion and this survey provides no evidence to justify regarding dysmenorrhea as a psychosomatic condition or as one calling for psychological treatment. In contrast, the syndrome of premenstrual tension seems to be very significantly correlated with neuroticism.

Renaer et al. (1959, unpublished work) administered the Minnesota multiphasic personality inventory (MMPI) to 20 young patients complaining of severe primary dysmenorrhea and 20 young women of the same age who had no dysmenorrhea. This psychometric evaluation did not show any difference between the two groups.

Prill and Franz (1968) subjected 100 women with moderate to severe dysmenorrhea and a group of 50 without menstrual discomfort to five different psychometric tests:

1) The neuroticism scale from the Eysenck personality inventory (EPI)
2) The manifest anxiety scale (MAS) of Taylor
3) The manifest hostility scale of Siegel
4) The Saslow, Counts, and Dubois test, which evaluates the tendency to translate emotional experiences into somatic reactions
5) A study of a few other personality traits

In the dysmenorrhea group, a significant increase of the mean values for neurotic tendencies in the EPI, of anxiety in the MAS, and of the tendency to translate affective experiences into somatic reactions was found. The appearance of dysmenorrhea at the age of 25–29 years, a longer duration of the catamenial discomfort especially in the premenstrual period, and the presence of concomitant nongenital symptoms were all factors associated with significantly higher neuroticism scores and therefore pointing to a neurotic etiology. The authors acknowledge that their results are at variance with those of Coppen and Kessel, but note that the British authors had selected patients with dysmenorrhea in the strict sense, whereas their own series also included patients with premenstrual discomfort. It may be surmized that the different selection of patients explains to a large extent the different results. Prill and Franz found indeed that in persons with dysmenorrhea in the strict sense the neuroticism scores were lower than those of the other patients. They therefore agree that in the "pure dysmenorrhea" group the neurotic etiology of the disorder is less frequent.

The absence of convincing evidence for a psychosomatic explanation and the pathophysiology data reported earlier indicate that the pathogenesis of primary dysmenorrhea seems to lie in the realm of pathophysiology rather than of psychogenesis. However, as in every problem of chronic and recurrent pain, psychologic and psychopathologic factors certainly influence and modulate the pain experience. Reading and Newton (1977) compared primary dysmenorrhea and pain related to intrauterine devices (IUD) by means of a modified form of a Melzack's pain questionnaire. The word checklists were divided into four categories for scoring purposes: (1) words indicating sensory properties of pain, (2) words indicating affective properties, (3) words indicating evaluating properties, and (4) words giving temporal properties. IUD-related pain was expected to have a more prominent sensory component, as the presence of an IUD constitutes a tangible, known stimulus produced by a useful object. It was expected, on the other hand, that dysmenorrhea would give rise to greater distress owing to its unavoidable nature. The study showed that there was little difference between the degree of pain in each group, but it appeared that women with dysmenorrhea report more affective words, denoting distress and emotional reaction, while IUD users with severe pain report a greater number of sensory words.

8.3.3.2 A Pathophysiologic Explanation

The finding of some divergence in the clinical course of dysmenorrhea and of some variability in the parameters of the uterine contractions, as well as the lack of uniformity in the results obtained by some specific treatment methods (see below), indicate that apparently not all cases of primary dysmenorrhea share the same pathogenetic mechanism. More pathophysiologic data are necessary. Meanwhile, the most important factors whose interaction is thought to determine the pain experience of primary dysmenorrhea will be emphasized.

Hypertony of the uterine isthmus on the day before and on the 1st day of the period, as observed by Palmer and Liesse, by Youssef, and by Mann, seems to play a role in as many as 70% of the patients according to Mann. The tracings of Filler and Hall (their Fig. 3) indicate that in some cases it is not so much the absolute value of the intrauterine pressure but the pressure exercised by the uterine contents on the abundantly innervated and tight isthmus, which determines the cramplike pain. The menstrual tracings of most authors, however, tend to show that in most cases the pain is associated with spastic or dysrhythmic contractions combined with high basal tones; this pattern may cause pain by provoking myometrial ischemia. At this time, the respective role of these two pain mechanisms (pressure on the isthmus and myometrial ischemia) is not known; moreover, the cause of the premenstrual and menstrual isthmic hypertony found in many cases remains to be elucidated.

The high prostaglandin content of the endometrium on the 1st day of the period seems to determine the contractility patterns associated with most cases of primary dysmenorrhea. Whereas there is no difference in the endometrial prostaglandin content of dysmenorrheic and nondysmenorrheic women during the premenstrual period, the content of the menstrual endometrium is significantly higher in most dysmenorrheic patients; this may be the result of a disturbed outflow of menstrual blood through the cervix (Moghissi 1972; Åckerlund 1979). As will be mentioned later, various recent treatment methods, when efficacious, cause a decrease in the prostaglandin content of the menstrual endometrium, correlated with a decrease in the basal tone and in the intensity of the contractions and accompanied by a disappearance of the spastic contractions.

Further advances in research on the pathogenesis of primary dysmenorrhea are likely to be obtained by discarding cases that do not correspond to a strict definition of the disorder and by correlating the clinical characteristics with the radiologic, biophysical, and biochemical parameters described above.

8.3.4 Management

The method of treatment will depend on the severity of the condition and on a number of actual circumstances. Is the patient married or single? Is she prepared to take "the pill" for months or years? Is it important for her never to cut classes or to miss work?

Detailed information concerning the characteristics of the dysmenorrhea and a careful clinical examination will be helpful in verifying that the patient has a primary or essential dysmenorrhea.

The patient and her mother should be told that there is nothing seriously wrong with either the structure or function of the genital organs, that the pain, paradoxically, gives evidence that her ovarian function is normal, and that although the condition is not easily cured, there certainly is a possibility to help her. She may also be told that she has an 80%–90% chance of getting rid of her pain with the birth of her first baby. The fact that good results are reported in a percentage of the patients by reassurance alone has been interpreted by some authors as proof of the psychogenic origin of the disorder. There is, however, no comparison between the results obtained by psychotherapy and those obtained in double-blind therapeutic experiments with drugs whose mode of action is based on the pathophysiologic mechanisms described above.

8.3.4.1 Medical Treatment

Mild forms may be treated by analgesics or antispasmodic drugs supplemented by a mild dose (e.g., 15 mg) of codeine. Care should, however, be taken not to prescribe morphium derivatives or other habit-forming drugs for a condition that may recur during several years.

For severe dysmenorrhea, there is a whole spectrum of drugs that will procure symptomatic relief. Apart from a delivery or a presacral neurectomy, there is at present no treatment that cures the condition. From a pathogenetic point of view, the problem is how to influence the menstrual hypertony of the isthmus, the strong or the spastic uterine contractions with high basal tone, or the prostaglandin content of the menstrual endometrium that causes the contractions.

There have been a few attempts at influencing the isthmic tone by means of intravaginal administration of bromelain, which seems to widen the isthmus, but these studies have not led to practical applications.

Ovulation Inhibitors. It has been known since the early 1940s (Sturgis and Albright) that estrogens administered during the first 20 days of the cycle in doses sufficient to inhibit ovulation will prevent the pain of the next period. Since the late 1950s, estrogens have been replaced for the purpose of inhibiting ovulation by combined estroprogestrogens, prescribed in a cyclic manner. They provide symptomatic relief, as long they are taken, in eight or nine of ten patients. Patients who are not helped by this cyclic therapy should be further investigated as their pain probably has either a structural or a psychogenic origin. Sequential drugs are less effective than combined estroprogestogens. Pressure waves with low frequencies, low basal pressures, and moderate amplitudes were seen under combined pills; there was, furthermore, no substantial difference between the effect of the combined pills and a mere progestational agent, such as lynestrenol, administered continuously in a dose of 5 mg a day starting on the 1st day of a period (Eskes et al. 1970; Hein et al. 1973). The prostaglandin content of the menstrual endometrium was greatly reduced after a cycle on combined pills as compared to the content after an untreated cycle (Lundström and Green 1978). It would thus seem that the therapeutic effect of the pills is mediated by a reduction of the prostaglandin content of the endometrium. In continental Europe, some gynecologists prefer to suppress ovulation and menstruation by the continuous administration of a progestrogen, e.g., ethinyl estrenol (lynestrenol) or 5 mg of norethisterone acetate daily, starting on the 1st day of a period and continuing for several months or years. These steroids may, however, cause obesity and sometimes loss of libido.

Some patients also have, besides their dysmenorrhea, a problem of infertility and can therefore not be helped by ovulation inhibitors. They may be given 10 mg of retroprogesterone (Duphaston) twice daily from day 5–25 of the cycle (Bishop 1961; Fairweather 1965; Aydar and Coleman 1965). This drug is said not to interfere with ovulation, and recordings of the uterine contractions are approximately identical with those of a normal ovulatory cycle (Eskes et al. 1970).

Tocolytic Agents. The stimulation of β_1- and β_2-rexeptors, which are present in the myometrium, causes myometrial relaxation. It was therefore logical to try β-

receptor stimulators in dysmenorrhea. Baumgarten et al. (1969) obtained good results with ritodrine administered either orally or intravenously, but Hansen and Secher (1975) did not obtain good therapeutic effects with orally administered hydroxyphenylorciprenaline (fenoterol) compared to a placebo. On the other hand, terbutaline, a selective β_2-stimulator, given intravenously in doses of 0.25–0.5 mg on the 1st day of menstruation, inhibited myometrial activity, increased myometrial blood flow, and relieved the pain (Åckerlund et al. 1976). When terbutaline was given orally (2.5 mg three times daily), several patients were relieved of their pain, but they stopped taking the drug because of the side effects, the chief of which was tremor. Because of their side effects (tachycardia and tremor), the tocolytic agents have up to now had but a limited use in dysmenorrhea.

Prostaglandin Inhibitors. According to a dozen or so recent papers, prostaglandin inhibitors and antagonists appear more promising (Ylikorkala and Dawood 1978; Andersson et al. 1978; Kapadia and Elder 1978; Cornely et al. 1978). Indomethacin, naproxen sodium, mefenamic acid, and flufenamic acid have all been investigated, most of them in double-blind studies, and have been shown to give significantly superior results compared to the placebo-treated cases. Indomethacin has been studied more extensively than the other drugs; 25 mg of indomethacin given orally two to three times daily, starting 1 day before the expected menstruation and continued until the 2nd or 3rd day of bleeding, has given good results and caused few side effects. The administration of these nonsteroid anti-inflammatory drugs is followed in most cases of primary dysmenorrhea by the disappearance of the spastic contractions and by the return of the uterine tone between contractions to a basal level. There are exceptions to this rule, so that as has been mentioned earlier, there is probably more than one kind of pain mechanism at work in primary dysmenorrhea.
Much more clinical experience with these drugs will be needed before it becomes clear which one should be preferred; it should, however, be pointed out that aspirin-like anti-inflammatory drugs should not be used before the beginning of the period in patients desiring to become pregnant.

8.3.4.2 Surgical Treatment

In the past, extensive dilatations of the cervix – up to Hegar 14 – were frequently performed, but these so-called dilatations may provoke tears of the isthmus, which may later predispose to isthmic incontinence during pregnancy. Furthermore, the result generally lasts only a few months; this is why they have almost completely been abandoned.
Before the introduction of the ovulation inhibitors, presacral neurectomy (Cotte's operation) was performed rather frequently. Most patients with severe dysmenorrhea are now relieved by ovulation inhibitors, and those who are not are likely to be poor candidates for the procedure. A Cotte's operation may be indicated for a patient with primary dysmenorrhea who does not tolerate ovulation inhibitors or for whom they are contraindicated.

8.4 Secondary Dysmenorrhea

A dysmenorrhea is called secondary if a structural anomaly is responsible for the pain; it generally occurs later in reproductive life than the primary variety; but there are exceptions. The most frequent causes will now be considered briefly.

8.4.1 Endometriosis

Secondary dysmenorrhea is a common symptom of endometriosis. This kind of menstrual pain is commonly thought to start in the late 20s or in the 30s, to last as long as the period itself, and to become gradually more severe over the years. These are indeed the clinical characteristics in a number of cases, but Chap. 11 stresses the different patterns that may be found in the pain symptoms.

During the last 3 decades, a great number of young patients have for diverse reasons undergone laparoscopies, and these examinations have revealed that endometriosis and the dysmenorrhea it may cause are much more common in women in their teens and early 20s than used to be assumed. This observation had already been made by Fallon (1946); it was emphasized more recently by Schiffrin et al. (1973) and by Gautier (1976) and is being verified in every center involved in the detailed work-up of infertility cases.

The diagnosis will be easy if the gynecologic examination reveals lesions suggestive of endometriosis, but as smaller lesions may not be palpated, we should suspect endometriosis when the pain lasts as long as the period itself or when it is unilateral or more pronounced on one side. It is insufficiently known that in some patients dysmenorrhea due to endometriosis presents with the clinical characteristics of primary dysmenorrhea. The true cause will be discovered when an examination under anesthesia or a laparoscopy is done in a patient whose "primary dysmenorrhea" does not respond to ovulation inhibitors. Parsons and Sommers (1978) state that 15% of the cases of incapacitating primary dysmenorrhea were found to have endometriosis at the time when surgical exploration and presacral neurectomy were more frequently performed. For the dicussion of the treatment, the reader is referred to Chap. 11.

8.4.2 Adenomyosis

In view of the similarity of the lesions with endometriosis (externa), adenomyosis has also been called endometriosis interna. However, owing to the differences in pathogenesis, clinical symptoms and signs, and therapy, it should be dealt with separately.

Since the clinical diagnosis of adenomyosis is rather difficult, it has repeatedly been called an elusive disorder (Emge 1962; Bird et al. 1972). In the great majority of cases, the diagnosis has to await microscopic examination of a hysterectomy specimen, but L. Emge has demonstrated that diagnostic accuracy can be enhanced greatly by paying attention to a few characteristic data.

The disorder is generally discovered in the 5th decade. It is frequently accompanied by other lesions. In an instructive review of 11 different papers, McElin and Bird (1974) found that adenomyotic uteri displayed, on average, leiomyomas in 50% of the cases, endometrial polyps in 7.3%, and endometriosis in 12.4%. The relative frequency of these associations explains the difficulty of distinguishing symptoms referable to adenomyosis from those resulting from concomitant conditions.

The *incidence* of adenomyosis, as found in 14 different series of consecutive hysterectomies, varied from 8%–70% (McElin and Bird 1974). This variability depends chiefly on whether the definition of adenomyosis is broad or strict and on the care taken to search for the penetration of endometrial tissue into the depth of the myometrium. Bird et al. (1972) seem to have made the most careful search, but on the other hand their criteria for calling a lesion adenomyosis were rather broad. For most authors, the pathognomonic feature of adenomyosis is the finding of endometrial glands and stroma at least one low-power field below the myoendometrial junction. Bird et al. also include what they call adenomyosis subbasalis, which is characterized by the presence of endometrial tissue within one low-power field below the basal endometrium; in so doing, they found an incidence of adenomyosis as high as 61.5% in 200 consecutive hysterectomies.

8.4.2.1 Symptoms

To differentiate symptoms due to adenomyosis from those that are not, Bird et al. (1972) studied a series of cases of "essential" adenomyosis, i.e., cases in which adenomyosis was the only reasonable symptom-producing factor. Of these patients, 64% complained of significant abnormal uterine bleeding, i.e., either menorrhagia or metrorrhagia; 28.3% complained of dysmenorrhea; 18.7% had both dysmenorrhea and menorrhagia. In some cases, pelvic pain not related to the menses may be found.

8.4.2.2 Diagnosis

The diagnosis is often difficult because adenomyosis is so frequently associated with fibroids. Symptoms and signs suggestive of adenomyosis are menorrhagia with or without dysmenorrhea in a parous patient who is in her 40s and has a moderately enlarged uterus. The enlarged uterus is firm and broad and, as the lesions are frequently diffuse, there are generally no well-circumscribed nodules, such as those found in a polyfibromatous uterus.

The uterine volume enlarges slowly over the years but rarely grows larger than a 14-week gestation. McElin and Bird (1974) ascribe great diagnostic importance to variations in consistency, size, and tenderness on palpation during the cycle, the size being larger and the tenderness more pronounced premenstrually. Estroprogestogens or continuous progestogens are less efficient in adenomyosis than in menorrhagias due to fibroids and in "essential" menorrhagias, i.e., those without obvious underlying pathology.

Some radiologists (Beclère and Fayolle 1961) have described hysterographic signs suggestive of adenomyosis. They are small diverticula of the uterine cavity, found either at the level of the fundus or along a lateral border of the uterus. The uterine cavity itself is not or only slightly deformed and certainly not as much as in the presence of fibroids. Most cases of adenomyosis will, however, not be recognized by radiologic means.

8.4.2.3 Treatment

Medical treatment by means of progestogens or estroprogestogens is not very rewarding. For diffuse adenomyosis, extending over the whole myometrium, a total hysterectomy is the treatment of choice. When dealing with a younger patient desiring pregnancy and with localized lesions, partial resection of the myometrium may be tried, but the prospects of fertility are very poor.

8.4.3 Fibroids

Although uterine fibroids are seen frequently, especially after the age of 30, it has been shown by König (1959) that they are only rarely responsible for dysmenorrhea. They may cause colicky pains and menorrhagias when they are extruded out of the myometrium into the uterine cavity and pushed against or through the cervical isthmus. If the uterine size is only slightly enlarged, a submucous fibroid or a fibroid polyp may be detected by hysterography. A circular or polycyclic filling defect of the uterine cavity due to a submucous fibroid is likely to deform the shape of the cavity, whereas a mucous polyp will not do so. Nevertheless, a dilatation and curettage or a hysteroscopy is necessary to conclusively differentiate a fibroid from a mucous polyp. Before attributing dysmenorrhea to a fibroid, it is advisable to look for other causes, among which the most frequent associated lesion is endometriosis.

When dysmenorrhea is due to a fibroid, treatment should be surgical. A fibrous polyp that is being extruded through the cervix will be removed by torsion. A myomectomy will be done for other fibroids if the woman wishes to maintain her reproductive potential and a hysterectomy if she has completed her family.

8.4.4 Obstructive Dysmenorrhea

Obstructive dysmenorrhea may be either a congenital or an acquired condition. Congenital atresia of the hymen or a transverse septum of the vagina and, very rarely, a congenital atresia of the cervical canal will give rise to a painful monthly cryptomenorrhea.

The dysmenorrhea due to a *congenital uterine and/or vaginal anomaly* is frequently unilateral. It may have its origin in a rudimentary uterine horn that does not communicate with the other half of the uterus. Right after the menarche, the pain will be due to retention of blood in the blind horn; later, it may partly be caused by foci of endometriosis developing around the fimbriae of the corresponding tube when retrograde menstruation has occurred for some months.

Unilateral dysmenorrhea may also be seen when one-half of a double uterus does not communicate with the vagina, i.e., when there is a one-sided cervical atresia.

Another cause is a uterus duplex bicollis with a septate vagina, one-half of which will give rise to a unilateral pseudotumor; later, the retained blood will cause a unilateral hematometra and finally a hematosalpinx.

Very rarely, a small tumor may be found along the lateral border of the uterus; after resection, it appears to be formed by uterine muscle surrounding a blind cavity filled with old blood. This is called a "müllerianoma."

In some cases of uterus duplex bicollis, the patient may complain of unilateral dysmenorrhea even without any obstruction; in such a case, the pain mechanism is probably the same as in primary dysmenorrhea.

It is important to remember that anomalies of the müllerian duct, and especially the asymmetric varieties, are frequently accompanied by anomalies of the wolffian ducts, such as absence or hypotrophy of one kidney.

Apart from the anomalies just mentioned, other forms are described by authors especially interested in these uncommon conditions (Jones 1977; Jones and Jones 1953; Jones and Whealess 1969; Rock and Jones 1977; Jeffcoate 1975; Müller et al. 1968; Musset et al. 1968a, b; Robert and Le Charpentier 1974).

The symptoms and signs of these congenital anomalies are very varied, as are the anomalies themselves. The presenting symptom may be either cryptomenorrhea, unilateral dysmenorrhea, dyspareunia, menorrhagia, or infertility. The diagnosis should rely first of all on history and on clinical examination. An early unilateral dysmenorrhea combined with the presence of an asymmetric mass in the lower abdomen or in the vagina is suggestive of an asymmetric malfusion deformity. Clinical examination may reveal either a double uterus or an unusually wide uterine fundus. However, other diagnostic techniques will have to be used to reach a complete understanding of the situation. A puncture of a blind vagina under aseptic conditions will reveal the presence of old blood; this puncture may be combined with the injection of an opaque medium to visualize the vagina and, indirectly, the uterus. A hysterography will also give important information. If any doubt remains, laparoscopy should be performed, as well as urologic exploration with intravenous pyelography; cystoscopy to explore the ureteral meatus may sometimes be desirable.

In view of the many different diagnostic and therapeutic problems that may be encountered in this field, the reader is referred to the papers especially devoted to this subject.

Acquired forms of obstructive dysmenorrhea may be due to adhesions in the cervical canal after an amputation of the cervix, a conization, or an electrocoagulation. Adhesions may also be situated in the lower part of the uterine cavity, e.g., in an Asherman syndrome after curettage for an abortion; they may also be a sign of a tuberculous endometritis. In both cases, the history will be very helpful. Hysterography will give an idea of the extent of the adhesions and, if a Novak curet can be introduced into the uterine cavity, histologic or bacteriologic examination of the endometrium may reveal endometrial tuberculosis. An Asherman syndrome will require either a dilatation of the cervix and lysis of the adhesions by means of a small blunt curet or a hysteroscopic resection. A genital tuberculosis will necessitate prolonged treatment with tuberculostatics.

We will not dwell here upon the so-called secondary dysmenorrheas, which are part of pain syndromes starting several days before the menstrual flow, such as a posterior parametritis that has developed on a chronic cervicitis, a "chronic salpingo-oophoritis," a so-called congestive dysmenorrhea, or "chronic pelvic pain without obvious pathology." These disorders or syndromes should not be classified as dysmenorrhea; they are therefore dealt with in other chapters.

8.4.5 Psychogenic Dysmenorrhea

The possibility of "psychogenic dysmenorrhea" will be raised if a patient with characteristics of primary dysmenorrhea or with a plausible cause of organic dysmenorrhea is not helped by means that are generally efficacious or if, apart from dysmenorrhea, there are other symptoms or a type of behavior pointing to a psychogenic origin of the complaints. However, we should only accept the diagnosis of psychogenic dysmenorrhea when no organic cause has been found and when a psychopathologic evaluation reveals a neurotic behavior or other psychopathologic problems. A patient with a probable diagnosis of psychogenic dysmenorrhea should be helped by symptomatic treatment and by psychotherapy.

It is, however, well to remember that the complexity of pain experiences is insufficiently accounted for by a simplistic differentiation into "organic," "pathophysiologic," and "psychogenic." This important principle should find its practical corollaries in any diagnostic evaluation and in the management of most patients with chronic or recurrent pain problems.

References

Åckerlund M (1979) Pathophysiology of dysmenorrhea. Acta Obstet Gynecol. Scand [Suppl] 87:27–32

Åckerlund M, Andersson KE, Ingemarson I (1976) Effects of terbutaline on myometrial activity, uterine blood flow and lower abdominal pain in women with primary dysmenorrhea. Br J Obstet Gynaecol 83:673–678

Andersson A, Haynes PJ, Fraser IS, Turnbull AC (1978) Trial of prostaglandin-synthetase inhibitors in primary dysmenorrhea. Lancet I:345–348

Andersson KE, Ulmster V (1978) Effect of nifedipine on myometrial activity and lower abdominal pain in women with primary dysmenorrhea. Br J Obstet Gynaecd 85:142–148

Asplund J (1952) Uterine cervix and isthmus under normal and pathologic conditions. Acta Radiol [Suppl] 91:3–76

Aydar CK, Coleman BD (1965) Treatment of primary dysmenorrhea: a double-blind study. JAMA 192:1003–1005

Baumgarten K, Seidl A, Fröhlich H, Sokol K (1969) Die Inhibition der Uterusmotilität intra menstruationem. Z Geburshilfe Gynaekol 171:145–158

Beclère C, Fayolle G (1961) L'hysterosalpingographie. Masson, Paris

Bengtsson LP, Theobald GW (1966 The effects of oestrogen and gestagen on the non-pregnant human uterus. J Obstet Gynaecol Br Commonw 73:273–281

Bird CC, McElen TW, Manalo-Estrella P (1972) The elusive adenomyosis of the uterus revisited. Am J Obstet Gynecol 112:583–593

Bishop PMF (1961) A new oral progestogen in the treatment of dysmenorrhea. Proc R Soc Med 54:752–574
Borell V, Fernström J (1953) Sphincter mechanism of isthmus uteri; radiological study. Acta Obstet Gynaecol Scand 32:7–12
Browne OD (1949) A survey of 113 cases of primary dysmenorrhea treated by neurectomy. Am J Obstet Gynecol 57:1053–1068
Cibils LA (1967) Contractility of the non-pregnant human uterus. Obstet Gynecol 30:441–461
Coppen A, Kessel N (1963) Menstruation and personality. Br J Psychiatry 109:711–721
Cornely H, Beutnagel H, Schönhöfer PS (1978) Symptomatische Therapie der primären Dysmenorrhoe durch Prostaglandinsynthesehemmung mit Indomethacin. Geburtshilfe Frauenheilkd 38:18–24
Cotte G, Dechaume J (1931) Les plexalgies hypogastriques. Documents histopathologiques. Presse Med 39:373–376
Csapo AI, Pulkkinen MO, Henzl MR (1977) The effect of naproxensodium on the intrauterine pressure and menstrual pain of dysmenorrheic patients. Prostaglandins 13:193–199
Davis A (1938) Dysmenorrhea: its aetiology, pathology and treatment. Oxford University Press, London
Diehl WK, Hundley JM (1948) Role of uterine motility in essential dysmenorrhea. Am J Obstet Gynecd 56:281–290
Emge L (1962) The elusive adenomyosis of the uterus. Am J Obstet Gynecd 83:1541–1563
Eskes TKAB, Hein PR, Stolte LAM, Kars-Villanova EB, Crone A, Braaksma JT, Janssens J (1970) Influence of dydrogesterone on the activity of the non-pregnant uterus. Am J Obstet Gynecol 106:1235–1242
Fairweather DVI (1965) Duphaston in dysmenorrhea; the results of a doubleblind clinical trial. J Obstet Gynaecol Br Emp 72:193–195
Fallon J (1946) Endometriosis in youth. JAMA 131:1405–1406
Filler WW, Hall WC (1970) Dysmenorrhea and its therapy: a uterine contractility study. Am J Obstet Gynecol 106:104–109
Gautier PJ (1976) L'endométriose de la jeune fille. In: Merz WR, Rey-Stocker I (eds) Proceedings of the IIIrd International Symposium on pediatric and adolescent gynecology. Lausanne, pp 207–212
Halbert PL, Damas LM, Jones DED (1976) Dysmenorrhea and prostaglandin (Review). Obstet Gynecol Surv 31:77–81
Haman JO (1944) Pain threshold in dysmenorrhea. Am J Obstet Gynecol 47:686–691
Hansen MK, Secher WJ (1975) Betareceptor stimulation in essential dysmenorrhea. Lancet 1:345–348
Hauser GA (1960) Die Rolle des neurovegetativen Nervensystems in der Gynäkologie und Geburtshilfe. Fortschr Geburtshilfe Gynaekol 10:17–258
Hein PR, Eskes TKA, Stolte LAM, Braaksma JT, Janssens J, van den Hoeck JM (1973) The influence of steroids on uterine motility in the non-pregnant human uterus. In: Josimovich JB (ed) Uterine contraction. Wiley, New York, pp 107–128
Hendricks CH (1964) A new technique for the study of motility in the non-pregnant human uterus. J Obstet Gynecol Br Commonw 71:712–715
Hendricks CH (1966) Inherent motility patterns and response characteristics in the non-pregnant human uterus. Am J Obstet Gynecol 96:824–843
Jeffcoate TNA (1975) Principles of gynaecology, 4th edn. Butterworth's, London
Jeffcoate TNA, Lerer S (1945) Hypoplasia of uterus with special reference to spasmodic dysmenorrhea. J Obstet Gynaecol Br Emp 52:97–121
Jones HW (1977) Surgery of the double uterus. In: Mattingly R (ed) The Linde's operative gynecology. Lippincot, Philadelphia, pp 309–319

Jones HW, Jones JS (1953) Double uterus as an etiologic factor in repeated abortion: indication for surgical repair. Am J Obstet Gynecol 68:325–339

Jones HW, Wheales CR (1969) Salvage of the reproductive potential of women with anomalous development of the müllerian ducts, 1868–1968–2068. Am J Obstet Gynecol 104:348–364

Kapadia L, Elder MG (1978) Flufenamic acid in treatment of primary spasmodic dysmenorrhea. Lancet 1:348–350

König PA (1959) Statistischer Beitrag zum Dysmenorrhoe-Problem. Arch Gynaekol 192:174–191

Lackner JE, Krohn L, Soskin S (1937) Etiology and treatment of primary dysmenorrhea; physiologic and clinical study. Am J Obstet Gynecol 34:248–266

Lennane KJ, Lennane RJ (1973) Alleged psychogenic disorders in women – a possible manifestation of sexual prejudice. N Engl J Med 288:288–292

Liesse AC (1947) Les dysmenorrhées fonctionnelles. Conceptions physiopathologiques. Rev Fr Gynécol 42:29–38

Lukas KH (1965) Die Dysmenorrhoe. Enke, Stuttgart

Lundström V, Green K (1978) Endogenous levels of prostaglandin F_{2a} and its main metabolites in plasma and endometrium of normal and dysmenorrheic women. Am J Obstet Gynecol 130:640–646

Lundström V, Green K, Wiqvist N (1976a) Prostaglandins, indomethacin and dysmenorrhea. Prostaglandins 11:893–907

Lundström V, Wiqvist N, Green K (1976b) Prostaglandins and dysmenorrhea. In: Samuelsson B, Paoletti R (eds) Advances in prostaglandin and thromboxane research, vol 2. Raven, New York, pp 996

Mann EC (1963) Primary dysmenorrhea. In: Meigs JV, Sturgis SH (eds) Progress in gynecology, vol IV. Grune & Stratton, New York, pp 123–145

McArthur JW (1957) Adolescent menstrual disorders. In: Meigs JV, Sturgis SH (eds) Progress in gynecology, vol 3. Grune & Stratton, New York, pp 58–79

McElin TW, Bird CC (1974) Adenomyosis of the uterus. Obstet Gynecol Annu 3:425–442

Moawad AH, Bengtsson LP (1967) In vivo studies of the motility patterns of the nonpregnant human uterus. I. The normal menstrual cycle. Am J Obstet Gynecol 98:1057–1064

Moawad AH, Bengtsson LP (1968) In vivo studies of the motility patterns of the nonpregnant human uterus. III. The effect of anovulatory pills. Am J Obstet Gynecol 101:473–478

Mocquot P, Musset R (1949) Remarques sur la physiologie pathologique des endométrioses a propos de 3 observations d'endométriose du cul de sac postérieur du vagin. Gynécol Obstét 48:134–154

Moghissi KS (1972) Prostaglandins in reproduction. Obstet Gynecol Annu 1:297

Moir C (1934) Intrinsic dysmenorrhea. Proc R Soc Med 29:950

Müller P, Musset R, Netter A, Dellenbach P, Hersat E, Dreyfus J, Koller B, Gillet JY (1968) Les malformations associées génitales et urinaires chez la femme et le problème particulier posé par les uterus cloisonnés. Gynécol Pra 6:453–479

Musset R, Müller P, Netter A, Sokol R, Trévoux R, Vinourd JC, Gillet JY, Poitout P (1968a) Les uterus communicants. Gynecol Prat 6:481–493

Musset R, Netter A, Müller P, Sokol R, Trévoux R, Vinourd JC, Gillet JY, Poitout P (1968b) Les accidents de retention menstruelle unilatérale observés en cas d'uterus malformés. Gynecol Prat 6:494–513

Palmer R, Palmer E (1963) Les explorations fonctionelles gynécologiques. Masson, Paris

Parsons L, Sommers SC (1978) Gynecology. Saunders, Philadelphia London

Pickless RV (1967) The prostaglandins. Biol Rev 42:624–652

Pickless RV (1979) Prostaglandins and dysmenorrhea. Historical survey. Acta Obstet Gynecol Scand [Suppl] 87:7–12
Pickless RV, Hall WJ, Best FA, Smith GW (1965) Prostaglandins in endometrium of menstrual fluid from normal and dysmenorrheic subjects. J Obstet Gynaecol Br Commonw 72:185–192
Polyshuk WZ, Sharf M (1965) Culdoscopic findings in primary dysmenorrhea. Obstet Gynecol 26:746–748
Prill HJ, Franz H (1968) Zur psychogenen Ätiologie der Dysmenorrhoe. Geburtshilfe Frauenheilkd 28:866–874
Reading AE, Newton JR (1977) A comparison of primary dysmenorrhea and intrauterine device related pain. Pain 3:265–276
Robert HG, Le Charpentier D (1974) Les bifidités utero-vaginales asymmétriques avec ou sans rétention menstruelle unilatérale. J Gynécol Obstét Biol Reprod 3: 1235–1254
Rock JA, Jones HW (1977) The clinical menagement of the double uterus. Fertil Steril 28:798–866
Roemer H (1969) Das Sexualleben der Frau und seine Störungen. In: Käser O, Friedberg V, Ober KG, Thomsen K, Zander G. Gynäkologie und Geburtshilfe, vol II. Thieme, Stuttgart, pp 487–544
Schriffin B, Erez S, Moore JG (1973) Teenage endometriosis. Am J Obstet Gynecol 116:973–980
Skajaa K (1951) Abdomino-pelvic pain in females without structural or organic pathology: plexalgia hypogastria. Acta Obstet Gynecol Scand 30:21
Sloan D (1972) Pelvic pain and dysmenorrhea. Pediatr Clin North Am 19:669–680
Sturgis SH, Albright F (1940) Mechanism of estrogen therapy in relief of dysmenorrhea. Endocrinology 26:68–72
Svennerud S (1959) Dysmenorrhea and absenteeism; some gynecological and medicosocial aspects. Acta Obstet Gynecol Scand [Suppl 2] 38:1–116
Wilson L, Kurzrock R (1938) Studies on motility of human uterus in vivo, functional myometrial cycle. Endocrinology 23:79–86
Woodbury RA, Torpin RA, Child GP, Watson M, Jarboe M (1947) Myometrial physiology and its relation to pelvic pain. JAMA 134:1081–1085
Ylikorkala O, Dawood Y (1978) New concepts in dysmenorrhea. Am J Obstet Gynecol 130:833–847
Youseef AE (1958a) The uterine isthmus and its sphincter mechanism. I. The uterine isthmus under normal conditions. Am J Obstet Gynecol 75:1305–1319
Youssef AE (1958b) The uterine isthmus and its sphincter mechanism. II. The uterine isthmus under abnormal conditions. Am J Obstet Gynecol 75:1320–1332

9 Midcycle Pain

The majority of ovulations are painless; many women occasionally experience some discomfort in an iliac fossa or in the lower abdomen around the time of ovulation, but only 1%–3% of the patients of a gynecologic outpatient clinic consult for midcycle pain (Gueissaz 1947).

The term midcycle pain or mittelschmerz is to be preferred to "ovulation pain" because only in a percentage of all cases is the pain due to ovulation. Midcycle

pain is mostly found in younger women: 70% of Whartons's and Henricksen's group of 61 patients (1936) were younger than 20.
Midcycle pain will rarely take a severe form; mostly, it assumes a less severe, recurrent form.

9.1 Severe Form

Some patients experience, around the date of ovulation, a severe pain in an iliac fossa, lasting some 20–30 min and then gradually fading away. This short lived pain is probably related to ovulation. In the uncommon event in which ovulation is followed by an abundant intraperitoneal bleeding, abdominal meteorism will appear and sometimes shoulder pain and fainting. The abdomen is tender on palpation, but there is no muscle guarding. On the side of the bleeding ovary, the adnexum is particularly sensitive and so is the pouch of Douglas. In most cases, no fever is observed, and there is hyperleukocytosis only in the presence of severe intraperitoneal bleeding. If the pain is felt in the right iliac fossa, it is understandable that appendicitis is suspected and that an appendectomy is undertaken. Wharton and Henricksen stress the fact that an acute attack is frequently preceded by several episodes of mild midcycle pain.
The diagnosis of intraperitoneal hemorrhage from an ovulating follicle rests on the occurrence of the complication at the time of ovulation, the disappearance of the pain after a rather short acute episode, the absence of fever, and the absence of muscle guarding. Laparoscopy will resolve any doubt between an appendicitis and a bleeding ruptured follicle. The great number of unnecessary appendectomies performed in younger women (see Chap. 1) should at least have taught surgeons and gynecologists who, during an appendectomy, find a normal appendix to be aware of the possible presence of a bleeding follicle or corpus luteum, a focus of endometriosis, or other pain-provoking lesions in the pelvis.
The wall of the bleeding follicle should be sutured or, when a bleeding follicle or corpus luteum has to be enucleated, a careful ovarioplasty should be performed. To prevent postoperative adhesions, which might be detrimental to the patients's fertility potential, microsurgeons recommend taking great care of the hemostasis, meticulously approximating the borders of the ovarian wound, preferably with fine interrupted and inverted sutures, and making sure that all the blood is rinsed out of the pelvic cavity by means of a generous amount of Hartman's solution.
Fortunately, the severe forms of midcycle pain with intraperitoneal bleeding rarely recur. On the other hand, an ovary that has been sutured may subsequently become the origin of annoying recurrent midcycle pain.

9.2 Less Severe Forms

Recurrent midcycle pain may take the form of a twinge in the lower abdomen. Other patients feel cramps. The discomfort may last form a few hours to 1 or 2 days and, in some cases, up to 4 days.

The pain may be either unilateral or bilateral in the lower abdomen. It may be felt always in the same iliac fossa, alternately on one side and on the other, or in the whole lower abdomen. Frequently, it is accompanied by intermenstrual bleeding. Gueissaz (1947) found this association 52 times in 124 patients with midcycle pain. Wharton and Henricksen (1936) found it in 9 of 29 private patients with midcycle pain. This association is certainly more frequent in patients with midcycle pain than in control cases without pain (Papanicolaou 1933).

Midcycle pain generally does not present a great problem when it is short lived and not very severe. As long as neither the doctor nor the patient are aware of a recurrent character of the pain, it may be taken for appendicitis when it is right sided. The absence of nausea, vomiting, fever, and muscular rigidity on the one hand and the chronological relationship with the ovulatory period on the other should help to resolve the problem.

9.3 Pathogenesis

The different forms under which it may present itself prove that midcycle pain is not a disease but rather a syndrome, which may be due to various causes. There is a great lack of clinical observations to substantiate the pathogenetic explanations of midcycle pain.

If the pain is *unilateral and always on the same side,* it cannot always be directly related to ovulation, unless there is only one ovary left. In some such cases, it may be related to tubal pathology, e.g., a hydrosalpinx. Béclère (1947, cited by Gueissaz 1947) performed a hysterosalpingography on 15 patients with midcycle pain and found a bilateral hydrosalpinx in several of them. The pain may also be due to an ovarian or peritoneal focus of endometriosis, but these conditions are also apt to lead to dysmenorrhea. In some cases, the pain is always felt in the same iliac fossa but occurs only every second cycle. In others it occurs *alternately in the left and in the right iliac fossa.* Gueissaz found this alternate localization in 16 of 124 cases. In this situation, the pain seems directly related to ovulation, although it is not clear why the majority of ovulations remain painless. Only laparoscopy can show whether the pain might be caused by a perioophoritis, which impedes the expansion of the mature graafian follicle.

When the pain is *symmetrically localized* either in the hypogastrium or in the whole lower abdomen, there are several possible explanations, although it is difficult to ascertain which is the real one. It may be caused by an endometriotic focus situated in the pouch of Douglas. If the patient complains of cramping pains, it may be caused by the high basal pressure of the myometrial contractions (Filler and Hall 1970), which is indeed higher during the periovulatory period (Hein et al. 1973).

The pain may also be explained by the active congestion that occurs during the preovulatory estrogen peak. In a patient who had prolonged cycles and who complained of midcycle pain, Gueissaz artificially reproduced the pain by injecting 5 mg of estradiol dipropionate (Ovocyclin) several days before the customary date, and the spontaneous pain occurred a few days later at the expected date of ovulation. The hypothesis of pelvic congestion seems to be suggested by two sorts of considerations. We have observed a patient who during her periovulatory period regularly complained of spontaneous pain that exacerbated when she sat down. On examination, a rather large, sensitive uterus in mobile retroflexion was found. Furthermore, the relatively frequent coincidence of midcycle pain and midcycle bleeding is striking. The midcycle bleeding is most probably not an estrogen withdrawal, but a diapedesis bleeding due to a high estrogen peak; the two phenomena might thus, in some cases, have their common origin in an enhanced periovulatory uterine blood flow. It would, in fact, be interesting to determine the preovulatory plasma estrogen concentrations in a series of such patients and to compare them with a control group without bleeding and without pain.

9.4 Treatment

When the discomfort is mild, a prescription of analgesics will suffice and, if there is no history of pelvic inflammatory disease, the patient may be reassured that her ovarian function is normal. If the recurrent pain is more severe, the patient will be helped by cyclic estroprogestogens prescribed to inhibit ovulation.
Patients who desire to become pregnant and whose infertility checkup is negative may be prescribed 10 mg daily of methyltestosterone perlingually during 10 days beginning about 5 days before the expected date of ovulation.

References

Filler WW, Hall WC (1970) Dysmenorrhea and its therapy: a uterine contractility study. Am J Obstet Gynecol 106:104–109
Gueissaz E (1947) La crise intermenstruelle. In: Cotte G (ed) L'ovulation et ses troubles. L'Expansion Scientifique Française, Paris 118–134
Hein PR, Eskes TKA, Stolte LAM, Braaksma JT, Janssens J, van den Hoecke JM (1973) The influence of steroids on uterine motility in the non-pregnant human uterus. In: Josimovich JB (ed) Uterine contraction. Wiley, New York, pp 107–128
Papanicolaou GN (1933) Sexual cycle in the human female. Am J Anat 52:519
Wharton LR, Henricksen E (1936) Studies in ovulation. JAMA 107:1425–1432

10 Premenstrual Tension

Premenstrual tension is the name given in 1931 by Frank to a rather vague syndrome encompassing a host of disparate symptoms that appear in cyclic manner during 8-10/14 days before menstruation and disappear with the onset of the period.

10.1 Symptoms

The most common symptom is a generalized sense of distension felt chiefly in the breasts and in the abdomen. Many patients also complain of nervous tension, emotional instability, anxiety, and depression; some have tremor, dizziness, or insomnia.

Many patients are really disturbed as they feel they are difficult to get along with during their premenstrual period or because they fear they may be heading toward a nervous breakdown or a psychosis. Premenstrual tension causes generalized abdominal discomfort with bloating rather than pain. Therefore, and because the symptoms occur in the premenstrual and not during the menstrual period, it should not be considered a form of dysmenorrhea. Premenstrual tension may occasionally be accompanied by lower abdominal pain, but if there is pain in the lower abdomen, a cause other than premenstrual tension should be sought.

The number and the intensity of the symptoms vary from one cycle to another, and a period of several months with severe cyclic episodes of premenstrual tension may alternate with another during which the situation is much more bearable. Such spontaneous fluctuations render the evaluation of any particular treatment difficult.

10.1.1 Signs

The paucity of objective signs contrasts with the great number of symptoms. During the premenstrual period, the breasts are tender on palpation; the upper half has generally a firmer consistency than the lower, and the upper and outer part of both breasts may be more nodular. Sometimes a broad, poorly defined lump may be felt in the upper half or in the upper outer quadrant. To make sure that these signs are cyclic rather than constant phenomena, the patient should be reexamined during the 2 weeks following the end of the period. In fact, all breast examinations should preferably be performed at that time of the cycle (Haagensen 1974). Abdominal bloating is more a symptom than a sign as it cannot be objectivized on palpation.

10.1.2 Prevalence

The syndrome is most frequently seen over the age of 30. Its prevalence depends on the definition used, as has been shown by Sutherland and Stewart (1965). They gave a questionnaire to 100 university students and to 50 registered nurses. The mean age of these women was 21.9 years and only 3 were married. If the premenstrual or cyclic tension was defined as "irritability and depression," 53% of the persons questioned had it, whereas only 38.7% suffered from the triad "irritability, depression, and swelling."

10.1.3 Pathophysiology

Several authors have tried to find a histopathologic explanation for the fullness and tenderness of the breasts (Southam and Gonzaga 1965). Haagensen (1971) could not find in the breasts any histologic features characteristic of the premenstrual phase. However, the premenstrual engorgement of the breast – which is probably more pronouned in patients with premenstrual tension – must be due to blood and lymph engorgement or to an increase in extracellular fluid tension, which is difficult to demonstrate by routine microscopic techniques. It is generally thought that cyclic retention of fluid in the premenstruum is the most important factor in the pathogenesis of the syndrome.
A correlation between negative affect, weight, and urinary K/Na values has been found by Janowski et al. (1973) in normal college-age volunteers during the menstrual cycle. An increase in all variables was noted during the luteal and premenstrual phases of the cycle. These variables rapidly decreased around the time of the menses. However, several authors have reported cases of premenstrual tension without significant premenstrual weight gain (Thorn et al. 1938; Chesley and Hellman 1957). Bruce and Russell (1962) followed during 4–9 weeks the weight changes and the water, sodium, and potassium balance throughout the menstrual cycle in ten patients who had a constant food and water intake in a uniform environment. In four of ten, there was a distinct weight gain during the second half of the cycle, but in none of these four patients was there an increase in symptoms. In general, there was no good correlation between weight gain, water and sodium retention, and accentuation of the symptoms. This conclusion was confirmed by the findings of Golub et al. (1965) on the weight changes observed in 69 college women during their menstrual cycle. Andresch et al. (1978) followed the body weight, total body potassium, and total body water of 19 patients with premenstrual tension of at least 6 months duration and of 20 healthy women with no premenstrual symptoms. In neither group was there an increase in total body water. There was, however, a higher water/potassium rate in women with premenstrual tension than in control women, the difference being significant in the late luteal phase. The absence of significant weight gain suggests that some symptoms of premenstrual tension may be due to redistribution of fluid rather than to an increase in total body fluids. Recently, O'Brien et al. (1979) did not find a significant difference in the premenstrual weight gain of 18 symptomatic compared to 10 asymptomatic patients.

10.2 Pathogenesis

10.2.1 Premenstrual Tension and Personality

Coppen and Kessel (1963) examined the prevalence of dysmenorrhea and premenstrual tension in the general population and their relationship to personality. A questionnaire concerning menstrual symptoms was administered together with the Maudsley personality inventory (MPI) to a sample of 500 women of menstrual age. The MPI gives two measures of personality: neuroticism and extraversion. Neuroticism is defined as a general emotional lability of the personality, its emotional overresponsiveness, and its liability to neurotic breakdowns under stress. They found that certain symptoms (irritability, depression, tension headache, and body swelling) clustered together in a temporal relationship. These symptoms, which conform to the definition of the premenstrual syndrome, were most severe 1 or more days before the period. Moderate to severe degrees of the syndrome occurred in 25% of all women. The symptoms constituting the syndrome were significantly correlated with neuroticism, whereas dysmenorrhea, defined as pain during menstruation, was not. They also found that a woman who complained of premenstrual irritability was more likely to be irritable at other times as well.

It may therefore be assumed that the psychological symptoms of premenstrual tension are an exacerbation of personality traits that are related to neuroticism. In another paper on "The Prevalence of Menstrual Disorders in Psychiatric Patients," Coppen (1965) found that in neurotic patients, the symptoms of depression, anxiety, nervousness, and tension were much more frequent during the premenstrual and menstrual periods than in a control group. The results of Coppen and Kessel were confirmed and extended by James and Pollitt (1974). These authors studied the association between personality traits and the frequency, nature, and severity of premenstrual symptoms in 115 women, two-thirds of whom were psychiatric outpatients. The symptoms recorded were headache, tension or irritability, emotional lability, depression or elation, abdominal swelling, breast symptoms, and sleep disturbances. As the patients were questioned concerning 7 symptoms the total symptom score varied between 0 and 7. An estimate of the severity of the symptoms by grading each of them from 1 to 3 provided a weighted score for each symptom; the sum of the weighted scores was referred to as the "complaints score." Personality was assessed by using the self-rating hysteroid obsessoid questionnaire (HOQ) of Caine and Hope (1967). There was a significant correlation between the deviation from mean HOQ scores for each patient and her symptom and complaint scores. This suggests that the tendency to develop the syndrome is related to personality type and especially to extremes of obessionality and hysterical tendencies rather than to one specific personality type.

As there is a covariation between the symptoms of premenstrual tension and the function of the corpus luteum, the question has been raised whether premenstrual tension is not a behavioral disturbance conditioned by endocrinologic factors (Beach 1975). Possibly so, but before proposing a mediating mechanism, one should clearly establish what kind of change in mood or behavior one is studying and with which hormonal changes it is supposed to be correlated (Parlee 1973). If it is supposed that there is not only a correlation between premenstrual tension and progesterone secretion but also a causal relationship, the conclusion of a critical review by Glick and Bennett (1974) is all but encouraging: "the role of progesterone and the progestins in producing mood and behavior changes is still largely unknown."

10.2.2 Hyperestrogenism or Deficient Luteal Function?

Frank (1931) assumed that excess secretion of estrogens affecting thc sympathetic and cardiovascular systems was the cause of premenstrual tension. Others believed, on the basis of endometrial biopsies and curetting, that the syndrome was due to a relative deficiency of the corpus luteum function. None of these hypotheses has been confirmed by subsequent work (Henriksen 1962; Prill and Krüger 1963). Adamopoulos et al. (1972) assessed the pituitary and ovarian function of eight patients suffering from premenstrual tension by measuring their daily urinary output of total gonadotropic activity, estrogens, and pregnanediol. They did not find any major abnormalities in the endocrine functions examined but they did find, contrary to traditional belief, that premenstrual tension can exist in the presence of cycles with anovulatory hormonal patterns.

10.2.3 Hyperaldosteronism?

Gray et al. (1968) first described the increase of aldosterone secretory rates during the luteal phase of the normal cycle. Sundsfjord and Ackvaag (1970) reported significant increases in mean aldoterone excretion and plasma angiotensin II concentration of 100% and 75%, respectively. They suggested that the changes observed in concentration and excretion of these hormones was related as follows: the sodium-losing effect of progesterone stimulates renin activity, giving an increased plasma angiotensin II, which in turn leads to an augmented aldosterone production. It was therefore hypothesized that premenstrual tension might be due to a transient hyperaldosteronism. However, this seems improbable: primary hyperaldosteronism, although giving rise to excess salt and fluid retention, is not accompanied by the mood changes that are frequently seen in premenstrual tension. In an experiment designed to throw light on the pathogenesis as well as treatment, O'Brien et al. (1979) devised visual analogue scales for eight common mood types: depression, sadness, tension, feeling of bloatedness, loss of libido, aggression, lethargy, and anxiety. The subjects marked a 100 mm scale for each mood type at the same time each day, at a point along the line they felt appropriate to their mood. The score was determined by measuring the distance in millimeters, this being proportional to symptom change. The total score was calculated for each day. The difference between the preovulation and the premenstrual phase mean gave the premenstrual mood index (PMI); a positive score indicated a symptomatic cycle. Twenty-eight subjects were studied in a double-blind crossover trial of spironolactone therapy. The subjects' cycles were divided into menstrual, preovulatory, postovulatory, and premenstrual phases. Blood samples taken in each phase of the first two cycles were assayed for progesterone and aldosterone. Only those with a positive premenstrual mood index in all placebo cycles were considered the symptomatic group and those with inconsistent changes, the control group. Eighteen subjects were defined as symptomatic; ten belonged to the control group. the level of progesterone was significantly elevated in the symptomatic group during the postovulatory phase. There was a weak but significant correlation between the PMI and the postovulatory progesterone level. There was a significant rise of plasma aldosterone in the premenstrual phase of all subjects, but the aldosterone level of the symptomatic group was lower, although not significantly lower, than that of the control group. There was no significant correlation between the PMI and the premenstrual aldosterone level. It follows that premenstrual tension does not seem to be due to hyperaldosteronism; it is possible that progesterone in some way influences premenstrual tension symptoms. The authors feel that the syndrome is probably of multiple hormonal etiology.

10.2.4 Does Prolactin Play a Role?

Horrobin (1974) suggested that prolactin may have a role in the pathogenesis of the syndrome. Halbreich et al. (1976) found that throughout the menstrual cycle the mean serum prolactin concentration is significantly higher in women with premenstrual tension than in controls. They wondered, however, whether the increase in the serum prolactin concentration is merely an indicator of stress or is involved in the pathogenetic mechanism of the syndrome.
Benedek-Jaszmann and Hearn-Sturtevant (1976) did not find a higher than normal prolactin concentration in patients with premenstrual tension. In ten women with premenstrual tension, 2.5 mg of bromocriptine was administered twice daily from the 10th day of the cycle in a double-blind crossover experiment. All showed a significant improvement in breast symptoms and mood with bromocriptine but not with placebo. Anderson et al. (1977) determined the serum prolactin levels on the 7th and the 26th days of three consecutive cycles in 21 patients with severe premenstrual complaints. The first cycle was the control cycle and the two others were either drug or placebo-treated cycles in a double-blind crossover manner. The mean levels of the 7th as well as of the 26th day were within the normal range, and none of the patients had a persistently elevated prolactin level. All the patients received 2.5 mg of bromocriptine twice daily from the expected day of ovulation until the start of the menstrual flow. The only significant difference in the effects of the drug and the placebo was on the breast pain.
There is thus no clear evidence that an anomaly in prolactin secretion causes premenstrual tension. This conclusion seems to be confirmed by the fact that in most cases of amenorrhea with hyperprolactinemia there are no symptoms of premenstrual tension.

10.3 Treatment

10.3.1 General Remarks

The pathogenesis of this condition not being known, treatment must be symptomatic. During 25 years, from 1936 to 1961, Henriksen (1962) tried 47 different treatment methods of drug regimens and observed good results with 43. This optimistic but somewhat disconcerting report seems to prove that the placebo effect of the drug or of the management has a great influence; in fact, this has been clearly shown in several double-blind treatment trials. To a large extent, the favorable results can probably be explained by the psychotherapeutic effect of a supportive doctor-patient relationship. Indeed, the very nature of the symptoms makes it imperative to listen attentively to the patients's problems and to examine her carefully as, for example, the recurrent pain in her breasts understandably increases her nervousness and worsens her depression.

Friedrich and Labrum (1974) rightly make the following recommendations for an objective evaluation of any therapy:

1) The studies must be of a double-blind nature
2) Selection of subjects and criteria of cure should be based on clearly defined symptoms
3) The study should last long enough to allow for the variations from cycle to cycle in the intensity of the symptoms
4) Only one treatment should be tried at a time

There are unfortunately few studies that fulfil these criteria.

10.3.2 Drug Treatment

10.3.2.1 Diuretics

Based on the hypothesis that the syndrome is due to water and salt retention, various diuretics have been tried. Metolazone (Zaroxolyn) (Werch and Kane 1976) relieved both physical and psychological symptoms when compared with placebos in women who were selected for weight increase of at least 1.35 kg. In a double-blind trial, chlortalidone (Hygroton) was shown to be no more effective than placebo. Morton (1959) obtained better results with ammonium chloride than with placebos in women on a high-protein diet.

The administration of 25 mg of spironolactone (Aldactone) four times a day from day 18 to 26 of the cycle (O'Brien et al. 1979) significantly decreased the incidence of premenstrual mood symptoms, probably acting through its diuretic action. It appeared to be at least as effective as metolazone, although in this therapeutic trial the patients had not been selected on the basis of weight gain.

10.3.2.2 Sedatives

Sedatives, for example, meprobamate (400 mg three times a day) or 5 mg of diazepam (Valium), twice a day, during the 7–8 days before the period are useful for nervous tension, anxiety, and emotional instability. Some authors have reported good results with lithium carbonate in some patients with premenstrual tension (Sletten and Gershon 1966). They recommend 300 mg three times a day; lithium carbonate therapy should not be combined with a low-salt diet.

10.3.2.3 Prolactin Inhibitors

Bromocriptine (2.5 mg two times a day) has proved efficient for the relief of painful engorgement of the breasts (Benedeck-Jaszmann and Hearn-Sturtevant 1976).

10.3.2.4 Hormones

Although no hormonal imbalance has been found as a causative factor, several authors have claimed good results with progesterone (Greene and Dalton 1953; Colin et al. 1978) or with ovulation inhibitors (Speroff et al. 1978). Others have reported relief of the symptoms with buccal androgens, such as 25 mg of methyltestosterone or methyldihydrotestosterone during the 10 days preceding menstruation.

References

Adampoulos DA, Loraine JA, Lunn SF, Coppen AJ, Daly RJ (1972) Endocrine profiles in premenstrual tension. Clin Endocrinol (Oxf) 1:283–292

Anderson AN, Larsen JF, Steenstrup OR, Svendstrup B, Nielsen J (1977) Effect of bromocriptine on the premenstrual syndrome. A double-blind clinical trial. Br J Obstet Gynaecol 84:370–374

Andresch B, Hahn L, Andersson M, Isakson B (1978) Bodywater and weight in patients with premenstrual tension. Br J Obstet Gynaecol 85:546–550

Beach FA (1975) Behavioral endocrinology: an emerging discipline. Am Sci 63:178–187

Benedek-Jaszmann LJ, Hearn-Sturtevant MD (1976) Premenstrual tension and functional infertility. Aetiology and treatment. Lancet I:1095–1098

Bruce J, Russell GFM (1962) Premenstrual tension: study of weight changes and balance water, sodium and potassium. Lancet II:267–271

Caine TM, Hope K (1967) Manual of the hysteroid-obsessive questionnaire. University of London, London

Chesley LC, Hellman LM (1957) Variations in body weight and salivary sodium in the menstrual cycle. Am J Obstet Gynecol 74:582–590

Colin C, Gaspard V, Lambotte R (1978) Relationship of mastodynia with its endocrine environment and treatment in a double-blind trial with lynoestrenol. Arch Gynaekol 225:7–13

Coppen A (1965) The prevalence of menstrual disorders in psychiatric patients. Br J Psychiatry 111:155–167

Coppen A, Kessel W (1963) Menstruation and personality. Br J Psychiatry 109:711–721

Frank RT (1931) Hormonal causes of premenstrual tension. Arch Neurol Psychiatry 26:1053–1057

Friederich MA, Labrum A (1974) Evaluation and preferred management of premenstrual tension – Pelvic congestive syndrome and allied states. In: Reid DE, Christian CD (eds) Controversy in obstetrics and gynecology, II. Saunders, Philadelphia London, pp 760–775

Glick I, Bennett SE (1974) Psychiatric effects of progesterone and oral contraceptives. In: Schadee RI (ed) Psychiatric complications of medical drugs. Raven, New York, pp 295–331

Golub LJ, Menduka H, Conly SS (1965) Weight changes in college women during the menstrual cycle. Am J Obstet Gynecol 91:89–94

Gray MJ, Strausfeld KS, Watanabe M, Sims EAM, Solomon S (1968) Aldosterone secretory rates in the normal menstrual cycle. J Clin Endocrinol Metab 28:1269–1275

Greene R, Dalton K (1953) Premenstrual syndrome. Br Med J I:1007–1014

Haagensen CD (1971) Diseases of the breast, 2nd edn. Saunders, Philadelphia London

Haagensen CD (1974) The role of the gynecologist in the differential diagnosis of benign abnormalities of the breast and early breast carcinoma. In: Reid DE, Christian CD (eds) Controversy in obstetrics and gynecology, II. Saunders, Philadelphia London, pp 467–488

Halbreich U, Ben-David M, Assael M, Bornstein R (1976) Serumprolactin in women with premenstrual syndrome. Lancet 'I:654–656

Henriksen E (1962) The melancholies of menstruation and premenstrual tension. Clin Obstet Gynecol 5:252–259

Horrobin DF (1973) Prolactin; Physiological and clinical significance. Medical and Technical Publishing, Lancaster

James H, Pollitt J (1974) Personality and premenstrual tension. Proc R Soc Med 67:921–923

Janowski DS, Berens SC, Davis JM (1973) Correlations between mood, weight, and electrolytes during the menstrual cycle: A renin-angiotensin-aldosterone hypothesis of premenstrual tension. Psychosomat Med 35:143–154

Morton JH (1959) Premenstrual tension. Clin Obstet Gynecol 2:136–152

O'Brien PMS, Craven D, Selby C, Symonds EM (1979) Treatment of premenstrual syndrome by spironolactone. J Obstet Gynaecol 86:142–147

Parlee MB (1973) The premenstrual syndrome. Psychol Bull 80:454–465

Prill HJ, Krüger E (1963) Über die Östrogenausscheidung bei Frauen mit prämenstruellem Syndrom. Endokrinologie 44:34–38

Sletten IW, Gershon S (1966) The premenstrual syndrome: a discussion of its pathophysiology and treatment with lithium ion. Compr Psychiatry 7:197–206

Southam AL, Gonzaga FP (1965) Systemic changes during the menstrual cycle. Am J Obstet Gynecol 91:142–165

Speroff L, Glass RH, Kase NG (1978) Clinical gynecologic endocrinology and infertility, 2nd edn. Williams & Wilkins, Baltimore

Sundsfjord JA, Aakvaag A (1970) Plasma angiotensin II and aldosterone excretion during the menstrual cycle. Acta Endocrinol (Copenh) 64:452–458

Sutherland H, Stewart I (1965) A critical analysis of the premenstrual syndrome. Lancet I:1180–1183

Thorn GW, Nelson KR, Thorn DW (1938) A study of the mechanism of edema associated with menstruation. Endocrinology 22:155–163

Werch A, Kane RE (1976) Treatment of premenstrual tension with metazolone: a double-blind evaluation of a new diuretic. Curr Ther Res 19:565–572

11 Endometriosis

The term endometriosis designates foci of endometrium that develop outside the endometrial cavity. Internal endometriosis or adenomyosis, which indicates ectopic foci in the depth of myometrium, is briefly dealt with under "dysmenorrhea."

Recent extensive reviews of the subject have been given by Varangot et al. (1965), Pollosson and Rochet (1965), Movers (1971), Chalmers (1975), and Greenblatt et al. (1976). This chapter will be limited to data useful for the diagnosis and interpretation of pain symptoms and their treatment.

11.1 Incidence

As many endometriotic lesions are symptomless or cannot be felt on gynecologic examination, the frequency with which endometriosis is found depends on the circumstances in which it is sought. Endometriosis is present in about 15% of all cases undergoing laparoscopy or laparotomy (Giraud et al. 1971). In a series of 200 consecutive laparoscopies, we found endometriosis in 31 cases; in the 108 cases in which the laparoscopy was done for chronic pain, we concluded after a complete diagnostic evaluation that endometriosis was the likely cause of the pain in 22 cases (20%). When pain was not the indication for laparoscopy, we found endometriosis in 9 of 92 cases (10%). Williams and Pratt (1977) found it, however, in 50% of 968 consecutive celiotomies. It used to be thought that endometriosis was most common in women in their 30s and 40s, but as more frequent use has been made of laparoscopy, many more cases have been found in younger women and in teenagers (see Chap. 8).

Table 6. Location of the lesions in 485 celiotomies in which endometriosis was found. Williams and Pratt (1911) Location of the lesions in 485 celiotomies in which endometriosis was found. Amer J Obs & Gyn 129:245–250

Location	No.	%
Female organs		
Ovary	266	54
Tube	33	7
Uterus	277	57
Pouch of Douglas	331	68
Gastrointestinal tract		
Rectosigmoid	172	35
Ileum	9	2
Appendix	17	3
Urinary tract		
Bladder	73	15
Ureter	7	1.5
Elsewhere	8	1.5

Table 6 gives the location of the lesions in 485 celiotomies in which endometriosis was found (in many cases there were two or more different foci) (Williams and Pratt 1977).

11.2 Diagnosis

It is estimated that of 100 patients with pelvic endometriosis, about 30% are asymptomatic. The most frequent symptoms are: dysmenorrhea, cyclic lower abdominal pain or continuous pain, pain on defecation during the menstrual period, infertility, meno- or metrorrhagia, and deep dyspareunia. Table 7, modified from Scott and Burt (1962), shows the relative frequency of the various symptoms of 398 patients operated for histologically verified endometriosis. No single symptom is pathognomonic, but some are highly suggestive.

Spontaneous Pain

It has frequently been stated that dysmenorrhea due to endometriosis is a late-onset variety, i.e., a variety that frequently begins in the late 20s or 30s, whose severity increases over the years, and is most pronounced at the end of menstruation or 1 or 2 days after its end. When this kind of dysmenorrhea is found, it is indeed very suggestive, but in 50 consecutive cases of endometriosis, we found this type only 10 times (20%) (Renaer 1971). In teenagers, menstrual pain due to endometriosis may mimic primary or essential dysmenorrhea.

Although secondary dysmenorrhea is an early symptom of endometriosis, in many cases the pain gradually extends from the menstrual into the intermenstrual period. Of our own 50 cases, 26 had continuous pain, with or without menstrual exacerbation. In 3 of 50 cases, there was pain exacerbation at the time of ovulation.

Dyspareunia is a common symptom. Of our 50 patients 10 had it, but not all the

Table 7. Complaints in 398 patients operated primarly for endometriosis (Scott and Burt 1962). Reprinted by permission from the Southern Medical Journal (55:129–136)

	No.	%
Pain unrelated to menses	180	45.2
Dysmenorrhea – primary increasing or acquired	138	34.7
Abnormal uterine bleeding	135	33.9
Dysmenorrhea – other than primary increasing or acquired	122	30.6
Infertility	58	17.1
Pain related to menses	48	12.2
Dyspareunia	32	8.0
Urinary tract symptoms	29	7.3
Gastrointestinal symptoms other than pain	21	5.3

[a] Totaling more than 398 and 100% because many patients had more than one complaint

patients were married. The dyspareunia is nearly always of the deep variety. It may be due to pressure either on an enlarged, adherent adnexum in the pouch of Douglas, on a fixed retroversion, or on sensitive uterosacral ligaments.

The frequency of *infertility* attributed to endometriosis varies from one published series to another. This variation depends on several factors, for example, the type of clinic (special infertility clinic or general gynecologic outpatient clinic) and the techniques used in the investigation. There is, moreover, some uncertainty concerning the influence on fertility of foci of endometriosis that do not involve the ovaries and the tubes (Garcia and David 1977; Hammond and Haney 1978; Buttram 1979); this difficult problem, however, lies outside the scope of this book.

Intermenstrual bleeding with or without menorrhagia is frequently considered a symptom of endometriosis. Abnormal bleeding is less common in younger than in older patients with endometriosis, but even in the 4th and 5th decade, it is hardly more frequent in patients with than in patients without endometriosis, as meno- or metrorrhagia is mostly due to coincident lesions, such as fibroids or endometrial polyps. In a few cases, however, ovarian endometriosis may interfere with ovulation and with corpus luteum function (Parsons and Sommers 1978; Brosens et al. 1978). Superficial endometriotic implants, which may sometimes be found on the cervix after electrocauterization of an erosion, may give rise to slight pre-or postmenstrual bleeding.

Pelvic examination may reveal small, sensitive, nodular lesions, either in the uterosacral ligaments or on the posterior surface of the isthmus and the uterine corpus; these small nodules are almost pathognomonic signs of endometriosis. Examination may also reveal on one or both sides tender, enlarged adnexa, which are either laterally adherent to the uterus or fixed deep in the pelvis. A rectovaginal palpation may be more efficacious than a vaginal one. If tender nodules are not palpated between menses, they are sometimes found more readily during menstruation. Other common findings are a sensitive fixed retroversion or a firm, nodular mass in the upper part of the rectovaginal septum. Speculum examination will sometimes reveal a blue-domed cyst in the posterior vaginal vault; this endometrial tissue may also perforate the vaginal wall and appear in the posterior cul-de-sac as a friable mass that causes intermittent or continuous bleeding.

In the last 20–30 years, *laparoscopy* has gradually come to be used more frequently to identify large endometriotic lesions and to detect smaller ones. When there is doubt about the true nature of a cystic tumor, it may be punctured and emptied as far as possible under laparoscopy. By so doing, a chocolate cyst may be recognized, and the content of other tumors can be examined cytologically. Laparoscopy will also allow the differentiation of endometriosis from acute or chronic pelvic inflammatory disease and the evaluation of the extension and functional importance of endometriosis in infertility cases.

11.3 Various Pain Localizations in Endometriosis

Endometriotic implants may cause visceral pain, parietal pain, referred pain of visceral origin, and pain radiations of somatic origin.

11.3.1 Visceral Pain

Bilateral adnexal endometriosis causes pain in the lower abdomen; unilateral foci cause pain in the corresponding iliac fossa. The pain is frequently felt also in the dorsal gynecologic pain zone. Occasionally, it may be felt in the sacrogluteal zone only. When there is a third-degree fixed retroversion of the uterus, the pain may sometimes be located at the level of the lower half of the sacrum.
Rectal pain on defecation and tenesmus during the menstrual period is more common than is generally mentioned in the literature. We found menstrual pain on defecation in 23 of our series of 50 patients with endometriosis. This symptom is only rarely encountered in ohter painful pelvic conditions. A large left-sided endometriotic mass may exceptionally cause subocclusion of the sigmoid colon, especially during menstruation. Retroperitoneal extension of endometriosis with its attendant fibrosis may cause ureteral obstruction, but again this is quite exceptional. By 1969, some 64 cases had been described in the literature (Bates and Beecham 1969).
In view of the great frequency of surgical sterilization, it is worthwile to quote the experience of Palmer (1970), who successfully treated several cases of endosalpingiosis of the proximal tubal stump by laparoscopic electrocoagulation. Endometriosis of the bladder is much less frequent than the rectal localization. A vaginal or abdominal hysterotomy for second trimester termination of pregnancy is a predisposing circumstance. Symptoms may be either severe pain and frequency of micturition during the menstrual period or pain and hematuria.
Foci of endometriosis in the upper vaginal wall are rare. They may be found in patients who have never been operated on, but also after a total hysterectomy; they are then due to intraoperative transplants from the uterine mucosa. They are exceptional in intact vaginal mucosa.

11.3.2 Parietal Pain

Endometriotic lesions may be present at the level of the umbilicus; they may also be encountered in laparotomy scars after a midrimester hysterotomy, a cesarean section, or a myomectomy. The uncommon perineal endometriotic implants may give rise to a great deal of pain and discomfort either during coitus, menstruation, or both.

11.3.3 Referred Pain of Visceral Origin; Somatic Pain Radiations

In our 50 cases, unilateral adnexal masses were rather frequently accompanied by referred pain in the anterior surface of the corresponding thigh. An adnexal lesion may also refer its pain to the lower back, along the dorsal part of the iliac crista.
Endometriotic lesions will exceptionally provoke a somatic pain radiation due to irritation of either the obturator nerve in the obturator fossa, of the femoral nerve in the groin, or of the sciatic nerve. A few cases of "cyclic sciatica" have

been described but in only four cases was definite involvement of the sciatic nerve proved (Head et al. 1962; Forrest and Brooks 1972). Head et al. and Forrest and Brooks were struck by the presence of an evagination of the pelvic peritoneum in the direction of the greater sciatic notch. The endometriotic focus was found at the bottom of this evagination. This has been called "the pocket sign," a term coined by Head et al.: the cyclic appearance of a sciatic syndrome should draw the attention to the possibility of an endometriotic invasion of the nerve.

11.4 Mechanism of Pain Due to Endometriosis

About 30% – some authors say more – of all endometriotic lesions do not cause any pain symptom. Large foci, e.g., large chocolate cysts, may develop without causing pain; conversely, small lesions may be responsible for severe pain. Indeed, the pain will frequently disappear by laparoscopic cauterization or surgical excision of the focus. These facts raise several questions.

11.4.1 Pain Mechanism

The microscopic picture of the endometriotic implants reflects, to a variable degree, the cyclic changes of the mucosa of the uterine cavity. In some cases, the picture of the ectopic endometrium is similar to that of the uterine mucosa. In others, a proliferative phase is found in an ectopic focus when the uterine mucosa shows a secretory phase, but rather surprisingly, the reverse may also be observed: a secretory phase in an ectopic implant, while the endometrium is in the proliferative phase. Several hypotheses have been formulated to explain this variability. Nieminen (1962), studying the cyclic changes of the vessels of ectopic implants, divided his 174 cases into two groups: (1) superficial foci and (2) foci buried in the depth of surrounding tissues. In the superficial lesions, cyclic vascular modifications were found more readily than in the buried ones. It seems therefore probable that the surrounding tissues, and especially a fibrotic capsula, hinder the cyclic transformation of the implants (Varangot et al. 1965).

According to Sturgis and Call (1954):

> ...the lesions directly beneath or on the surface of the peritoneum may expand outward and bulge into the peritoneal cavity; on the other hand, lesions buried deeply below the surface more likely call forth an enveloping response. This may be the most important aspect of the disease that determines whether or not there will be periodic pelvic pain.

This explanation is underscored by suggestive illustrations showing superficial, nonencapsulated lesions without pain and encapsulated foci causing pain. At the macroscopic level, this theory seems to be confirmed by the fact that endometriosis in a scar in the abdominal wall or in an episiotomy scar will provoke cyclic pain as long as the focus remains closed and will become painless when it breaks through its capsula and opens on the surface of the skin.

In most cases, the pain seems to result from an increase in intratissue pressure and, more seldom, from indirect or direct involvement of a nerve. Premenstrual pain and the uncommon pain at the time of ovulation in endometriosis cases are probably effects of proliferation or edema in the ectopic implant. Menstrual exacerbation, which may sometimes take the proportions of an acute abdominal emergency, seems to be due to desquamation and bleeding into a closed cavity. There are, however, clinical varieties of pain that remain unexplained, e.g., continuous pain without menstrual exacerbation.

11.4.2 Why Do Some Lesions Remain Painless?

Superficially situated or open lesions generally are not painful, but to explain the painlessness of many closed lesions, recourse must be had to hypotheses that are hard to prove or to disprove.

Endometriotic lesions may be painless because of a low density of afferent visceral nerves at the site of the implant. A focus may cease to be painful because the ectopic tissues become nonfunctional as, for example, after the menopause, or during the reproductive period because the lesions is "burnt out" (Sturgis and Call 1954; Jeffcoate 1975). This last event may result from a reduction of the blood supply due to progressive fibrosis of the capsula (Mocquot and Musset 1949). In many cases, the pain decreases during pregnancy – sometimes after an initial aggravation – and for some time after pregnancy. This has been ascribed to decidual transformation and necrosis of the foci (Kistner 1966), but McArthur and Ulfelder (1965) found necrosis in only 1 case of a series of 24 pregnancies. It is probable that during pregnancy, endometriosis may become painless by an expansion of the capsula and that after pregnancy, the patient may be free of pain for a variable period owing to decreased tissue responsiveness to hormonal stimulation.

Large chocolate cysts are frequently painless. This may be ascribed to a slow expansion of their volume or to a less pronounced capsula formation (Parsons and Sommers 1978) and, in some cases, to pressure necrosis of the ectopic mucosa. It should be noted, moreover, that every tarry cyst is not due to endometriosis; it may also be a hemorragic lutein cyst.

Even taking into account the proposed explanations, the fact remains that in many individual cases it is difficult to see why a lesion is painless in a patient and why a perfectly similar lesion provokes severe pain in another.

11.4.3 How to Know Whether a Pain Symptom Is Due to Endometriosis

As many instances of endometriosis do not cause pain and as the pain provoking ones are not easily differentiated from the painless, it follows that the mere presence of an endometriotic implant does not necessarily mean that it is responsible for the pain.

The following data may be helpful. The site of the lesion should roughly coincide with the pain localization. Attempts can be made to reproduce the spontaneous pain by pelvic examination; this will sometimes have to be repeated during menstruation, as the foci tend to be more sensitive at that time. A laparoscopy will show the extension of the process and whether it is pink or red, i.e., superficial and devoid of a capsula, or blue-black or withish and penetrating more or less deeply into the surrounding tissues. Whenever it can be done without risk, a therapeutic trial by electrocoagulation may give the solution. Eight times out of ten, the pain of endometriosis disappears or decreases under cyclic treatment with estroprogestogens or under continuous treatment either with estroprogestogens or with danazol, whereas these drugs are generally less effective in other gynecologic pain syndromes.

11.5 Acute Pain Syndromes Due to Endometriosis

Although acute abdominal pain due to endometriosis is rather uncommon, it seems worth mentioning the various acute or recurrent syndromes endometriosis may occasion.

11.5.1 Intestinal Stenosis and Obstruction

In Table 6 we saw that endometriosis of the bowel occurs frequently, having been found in some 40% of 485 celiotomies for endometriosis (Williams and Pratt 1977). Gray (1973) found 179 cases in some 1500 patients operated on for endometriosis. The disease process mostly involves the rectosigmoid and, less frequently, the appendix, the terminal ileum, and the cecum. Intestinal obstruction is rare; it was present in two cases of Gray. Intestinal stenosis is more common: symptoms of stenosis recurring during consecutive menstrual periods are very suggestive of stenosing endometriosis of the bowel. Stenosis or obstruction may occur after menopause, although this is rare. During premenopausal years and after menopause, the differential diagnosis with colon carcinoma may be difficult and may occasionally necessitate a intraoperative biopsy. This diagnostic and therapeutic problem has been dealt with in several papers: Kratzer and Salvati (1955), Boles and Hodes (1958), Macafee and Greer (1960), and Gray (1973).

11.5.2 Acute Pain Without Rupture of an Endometriotic Cyst

In a series of 90 consecutive cases of endometriosis, we (Renaer et al. 1963) found 10 patients who had an acute pain episode; this coincided mostly with the menstrual period. In 7 of those patients, no rupture was found of a cystic mass at operation. The diagnosis was based on history and clinical examination but chiefly on laparoscopy.

11.5.3 Acute Pain Syndromes Due to Rupture of an Endometriotic Cyst

In 90 consecutive cases of endometriosis, we found 2 instances of a ruptured chocolate cyst. Cavanagh (1960) observed 9 ruptures in 649 cases, Ranney

(1970) 13 in 350 patients (3.5%), and Pratt and Shamblin describe 37 cases (1970). Pregnancy and therapeutic pseudopregnancy seem to predispose to this kind of complication. In the absence of pregnancy, rupture of a tarry cyst mostly occurs during the secretory phase.

The rupture presents as an acute abdominal emergency with severe pain starting in an iliac fossa or in the lower abdomen. The patient has nausea. There may be signs of intraperitoneal hemorrhage; the pain spreads over the whole abdomen. Tenderness and sometimes muscle guarding are found either over an iliac fossa or over the entire abdomen. A vaguely delimited mass is frequently found in an iliac fossa; in many cases, the cervix is painful on mobilization. There is mostly low-grade fever, but sometimes it may be as high as 39 °C. There is a moderately elevated leukocytosis (10000–18000) and sedimentation rate.

The differential diagnosis with appendicitis, ectopic pregnancy, and acute PID is difficult. It will only be arrived at if a cyst was known to be present and if it has suddenly disappeared; in most cases, it will be made at laparoscopy. Surgical treatment is imperative.

11.5.4 Pseudoappendicitis

In 4 of our extended series of 90 consecutive cases of endometriosis, the acute abdominal condition presented as an appendicitis. As shown in Table 6, the appendix was the site of endometriosis in 17 of the 485 cases of Williams and Pratt. The diagnosis of appendicular syndrome due to endometriosis is practically impossible, except perhaps by laparoscopy. When episodes of "appendicitis" recur during consecutive menstrual Periods, one should suspect right adnexal endometriosis. "Appendicectomy, among other operations, is a frequent experience in the patient with endometriosis without relief of symptoms" (Sutler 1947). In 1938, Davis noted that appendectomy is frequently followed by dysmenorrhea. This has also been our experience, but it is in fact probable that in these cases an appendectomy has mistakenly been performed on the occasion of a severe episode of dysmenorrhea due to endometriosis.

11.5.5 Pseudoinflammatory Variety

Moulonguet (1929) found that endometriosis may cause a slight rise in temperature before and during menstruation. According to Jeffcoate (1975), intermittent pyrexia is found in at least 10% of the cases, and Richter (1974) found a slight pyrexia in 55% of 324 cases. It is therefore not surprising that the diagnosis of recurrent acute or subacute salpingo-oophoritis is sometimes made. In the presence of "recurrent salpingo-oophoritis," genital tuberculosis should be sought and if this search is negative, the patient may be treated 2 or 3 months with cyclic estroprogestogens. However, in cases with recurrent pyrexia, it is even better to perform laparoscopy to establish the right diagnosis.

11.6 Management of Endometriosis

Treatment of endometriosis may be either hormonal, surgical, or combined. It has to be individualized as it will depend on a variety of factors: the age of the patient, the stage of the disease, the problems associated with the condition (infertility, pain, or both).

Although there are still discussions concerning "hormonal versus surgical therapy," it seems that opinions are tending toward a consensus that hormonal therapy has its proper indications, while surgery has others. Due to the variable extent of the lesions, comparisons of therapeutic results can only be made between cases of comparable severity. This is the reason why several authors have classified the lesions in several stages (Beecham 1966; Acosta et al. 1973; Mitchell and Farber 1974; Ingersoll 1977). Everyone agrees that there is an urgent need for a unified staging system. Well-documented treatment recommendations are given in Reid and Christian (1974), by Ingersoll (1977), and Hammond and Haney (1978).

In patients who are asymptomatic, have minimal disease, and are not desirous of becoming pregnant, periodic examinations every 6 or 12 months will suffice. Young married patients should, however, be warned not to wait too long before trying to become pregnant as the disease proces is likely to extend over the years.

Mild cases (Acosta I) without an infertility problem should preferably receive hormonal therapy to inhibit the growth of the endometriotic foci. This treatment may consist of a "pseudopregnancy regimen" with parenteral or oral administration of estoprogestogens. Wilkinson and Mattingly (1974) give a survey of the preparations used and the clinical results obtained. In Europe, 5 mg of lynestrenol daily or 5 mg of norethisterone acetate daily, starting on the 1st day of a menstrual period and given continuously for months or years, have been in use on a rather large scale, their goal being to realize a hypoestrogenic amenorrhea (Ferin 1964). Although both the pseudopregnancy regimens and the progestrogen-induced hypoestrogenic amenorrhea give good symptomatic results in eight or nine out of ten cases, they generally do not cure the disease. Indeed, in a significant percentage of the patients, the symptoms are apt to recur a few months after the end of the hormonal treatment.

Cyclic estroprogestogens also give good results as symptomatic treatment, but as far as the inhibition of the process is concerned, their use seems to be less logical as they do not suppress menstrual desquamation.

During recent years, many papers have tended to imply that the effect of danazol, by inducing a "pseudomenopausal situation," may equal or perhaps surpass that of the pseudopregnancy schemes. The properties and clinical applications of danazol are reviewed in detail by Dmowski (1979). Danazol, which is a synthetic steroid, has strong antigonadotropic and mild androgenic and anabolic effects. Given in doses of 400–600 mg daily, there is a strong reduction of the plasma estradiol concentration; and plasma progesterone levels indicate anovulation. The endometrium becomes atrophic. Amenorrhea develops within the first 4–6 weeks, although there may be some irregular spotting. A control study using laparoscopy and histologic evaluation demonstrated that in mild endometriosis there was complete disappearance of the disease after 3–4 months of treatment. In women with moderate and severe endometriosis of varying degree, the length of therapy varied between 6 and 18 months; there was complete disappearance of the disease in some, but in most patients regression was incomplete. In such cases, ectopic endometrium was typically atrophic (Dmowski and Cohen 1975). A 3-year follow-up study of 99 patients treated with danazol revealed a recurrence rate of 39%; on the other hand, 61% of patients remained asymptomatic and had no pelvic findings suggestive of recurrence. In the same study, the corrected pregnancy rate after discontinuation of treatment was 83% for cases with mild endometriosis, 73% for moderate, and 37% for severe cases (Dmowski and Cohen 1978).

A verification of the therapeutic results and of the side effects by others, and hopefully a reduction in the price of the drug, will show whether its use constitutes a progress in the medical treatment of endometriosis, as the two studies just quoted, and another by Noble and Letchworth (1977), seem to show.

Patients with mild endometriosis who desire to become pregnant but who complain of pain may for a few months try to become pregnant before submitting to conservative surgery to increase their fertility chances. In the meantime, it may be useful to prescribe 5 mg daily of methyltestosterone perlingually during a few months; this treatment has a 75% chance of giving at least partial relief of their pain (Hammond et al. 1978). For infertility, due to mild lesions, with or without pain, very careful conservative surgery seems to give the best results. The aim of the operation will be to excise or fulgurate the foci, to peritonize them as far as possible, and when needed to reduce a retroversion. A presacral neurectomy may be indicated when the lesions are located in the pouch of Douglas (Ingersobl 1977; Hammond and Haney 1978; Buttram 1979). A preoperative trial with pseudopregnancy to increase the chances of conception or to make the excision of fibrotic foci easier has has not been shown to be very efficacious. It does not seem that a postoperative pseudopregnancy regimen is useful either, as most conceptions that occur after surgery do so during the first months or year after the operation. Only a controlled comparative trial between conservative surgery and induction of a pseudomenopause with danazol would be able to demonstrate the superiority of danazol, but "the success rate of surgery will be hard to equal or to surpass" (Buttram 1979).

Essentially the same treatment as described applies to the moderate (Acosta II) and the severe (Acosta III) cases of endometriosis that cause infertility with or without pain, but understandably the prognosis from the standpoint of both pain and infertility is distinctly influenced by the stage of the disorder (Acosta et al. 1973).

In stage III cases in whom either palpation or laparoscopy reveal a definite enlargement of an ovary, it is wise not to start trying a hormonal treatment but to explore without delay the tumoral adnexa, which may sometimes harbor a neoplastic process.

If the patient fails to conceive after conservative surgery, a therapeutic trial with danazol is indicated. As it is frequently impossible, especially in moderate and severe endometriosis, to excise or destroy all lesions, a percentage of the patients are inevitably exposed to the risk of a later reintervention.

For patients who complain essentially of pain, who are not or no longer interested in pregnancy, and for whom a hormonal treatment is undesirable for some reason, total abdominal hysterectomy with or without conservation of one or both ovaries will be the treatment of choice. Whether one or both ovaries will be saved depends on the extent of the invasion of the ovaries and the possibility of excising or cauterizing most or all of the endometriotic implants. When it is difficult to eliminate lesions on the bladder or bowel wall, a total radical hysterectomy is advisable. Whenever lesions persist in the pouch of Douglas or on the rectal wall, a presacral neurectomy may guard the patient against a recurrence of her pain. After radical surgery, there is no objection to the use of low doses of estrogens for the treatment of postmenopausal symptoms, although this medical treatment may sometimes stimulate remaining foci. In the latter case, any spontaneous or provoked pain will usually disappear after interruption of the substitution treatment.

References

Acosta AA, Buttram VC, Besch PK, Molinski LR, Franklin RR, Vanderheyden JD (1973) A proposed classification of endometriosis. Obstet Gynecol 42:19–25

Bates JA, Beecham CT (1969) Retroperitoneal endometriosis with ureteral obstruction. Obstet Gynecol 34:242–248

Beecham CT (1966) Classification of endometriosis. Obstet Gynecol 28:437

Boles LS, Hodes P (1958) Endometriosis of the small and larger intestine. Gastroenterology 34:367–380

Brosens IA, Koninckx PR, Corveleyn PA (1978) A study of plasma progesterone, oestradiol-17β, prolactin and LH-levels, and of the luteal phase appearance of the ovaries in patients with endometriosis and infertility. Br J Obstet Gynaecol 85:246–250

Buttram VC (1979) Conservative surgery for endometriosis in the infertile female. Fertil Steril 31:117–123

Cavanagh WV (1960) Endometriosis. Bull Sloane Hosp Woman NY 6:115–122

Chalmers JA (1975) Endometriosis. Butterworths, London Boston

Davis A (1938) Dysmenorrhea: its aetiology, pathology and treatment. Oxford University, London

Dmowski WP (1979) Endocrine properties and clinical application of danazol. Fertil Steril 31:237–255

Dmowski WP, Cohen MR (1975) Treatment of endometriosis with an antigonadotropin, danazol: a laparoscopic and histologic evaluation. Obstet Gynecol 46:147–154

Dmowski WP, Cohen MR (1978) Antigonadotropin (danazol) in treatment of endometriosis. Evaluation of postreatment fertility and three year follow up data. Am J Obstet Gynecol 130:41–48

Ferin J (1964) Hypo-estrogenic amenorrhea and/or sterility induced by lynoestrenol. Int J Fertil 9:29–34

Forrest JS, Brooks DL (1972) Cyclic sciatica of endometriosis. JAMA 222:1177–1178

Garcia Cr, David SS (1977) Pelvic endometriosis: infertility and pelvic pain. Am J Obstet Gynecol 129:740–743

Giraud JR, Haudebourg JP, Payard J, de Touris H (1971) Aspects cliniques de l'endométriose génitale. Bull Fed Soc Gynecol Obstet Fr 23:589

Gray LA (1973) Endometriosis of the bowel: role of bowel resection, superficial excision and oophorectomy in treatment. Am J Surg 117:580–587

Greenblatt RB et al (1976) Recent advances in endometriosis. Excerpta Medica, Amsterdam

Hammond CB, Haney AF (1978) Conservative treatment of endometriosis. Fertil Steril 30:497–509

Hammond MG, Hammond CB, Parker RT (1978) Conservative treatment of endometriosis externa: the effects of methyltestosterone therapy. Fertil Steril 29:651–654

Head HB, Welch JS, Mussey E, Espinosa R (1962) Cyclic sciatica report of a case with introduction of a new surgical sign JAMA 180:123–126

Ingersoll FM (1977) Selection of medical or surgical treatment of endometriosis. Clin Obstet Gynecol 20:849–864

Jeffcoate N (1975) Principles of gynaecology, 4th edn. Butterworths, London Boston

Kistner RW (1966) Current status of hormonal treatment of endometriosis. Clin Obstet Gynecol 9:271–291

Kratzer GL, Salvati EP (1955) Collective review of endometriosis of the colon. Am J Surg 90:866–869

Macafee CG, Greer HLH (1960) Intestinal endometriosis. A report of 29 cases and a survey of the literature. J Obstet Gynaecol Br Emp 67:539–555

McArthur JW, Ulfelder H (1965) The effect of pregnancy upon endometriosis. Obstet Gynecol Surv 20:709–733

Mitchell JW, Farber M (1974) Medical versus surgical management of endometriosis. In: Reid DE, Christian CD (eds) Controversy in obstetrics and gynecology. Saunders, Philadelphia London, pp 631–636

Mocquot P, Musset R (1949) Remarques sur la physiologie pathologique des endometrioses, à propos de 3 observations d'endometriose du cul de sac postérrieur du vagin. Gynecol Obstet 48:134–154

Moulonguet D (1929) Un cas d'endometriose de l'ovaire. Bull Soc R Belg Gynecol Obstet 28:688

Movers F (1971) Die Endometriose. Enke, Stuttgart

Nieminen U (1962) Studies in the vascular pattern of ectopic endometrium with special reference to cyclic change. Acta Obstet Gynecol Scand [Suppl] 41:1–81

Noble AD, Letchworth AT (1977) Preliminary observations on the use of danazol in endometriosis compared to estrogen/progestogen combination therapy. J Int Med Res [Suppl 3] 5:79–80

Palmer R (1970) Laparoscopy in diagnosis and treatment of endometriosis and pelvic adhesions. Ned Tijdschr Verloskd 70:293–296

Parsons L, Sommers SC (1978) Gynecology, 2nd end. Saunders, Philadelphia London, pp 957–997

Polloson E, Rochet Y (1965) Traitement de l'endometriose génitale. Bull Fed Soc Gynecol Obstet Fr 17:293–350

Pratt JH, Shamblin WR (1970) Spontaneous rupture of endometrial cysts of the ovary presenting as an acute emergency. Am J Obstet Gynecol 108:56–60

Ranney B (1970) Endometriosis II. Emergency operations due to hemoperitoneum. Obstet Gynecol 36:437–442

Reid DE, Christian CD (eds) (1974) Controversy in Obstetrics and Gynecology Saunders Philadelphia-London

Renaer M (1971) Chronische pijn in de Gynaekologische Praktijk. Stafleu, Leiden Chronic Pain in Gynecologie Practice

Renaer M, Caudron J, Romelaert G (1963) Acute abdominale toestanden in de gynaecologische praktijk. Tijdschr Gastroenterol 6:154–163

Richter K (1974) Untersuchungen von 324 bis zu 17 Jahren beobachteten Patientinnen mit histologisch erwiesener Endometriosis externa. Geburtshilfe Frauenheilkd 34:21–28

Scott RB, Burt JM (1962) Clinical endometriosis: fifteen years experience at University Hospital of Cleveland. South Med J 55:129–136

Sturgis SH, Call BJ (1954) Endometriosis peritonei. Relation to functional activity. J Obstet Gynecol 68:1421–1431

Sutler MR (1947) Endometriosis of the intestine. Surgery 22:801–805

Varangot J, Giraud JR, Bignon-Schnizer J (1965) Etiologie, clinique et pathologie de l'endometriose génitale. Bull Fed Soc Gynec Obstet Fr 17:239–292
Wilkinson EJ, Mattingly RF (1974) Medical versus surgical management of endometriosis. In: Reid DE, Christian CD (eds) Controversy in obstetrics and gynecology. Saunders, Philadelphia London, pp 650–659
Williams TJ, Pratt JH (1977) Endometriosis in 1000 consecutive celiotomies. Incidence and management. Am J Obstet Gynecol 129:245–250

12 Chronic Pelvic Inflammatory Disease

Pain due to chronic pelvic inflammatory disease (PID) may result from an inflammatory process at the level of the cervix and the pericervical tissues, from a salpingo-oophoritis, or from a process involving both levels at the same time.

12.1 Chronic Parametritis Due to a Chronic Cervical Infection

Although chronic cervicitis is not painful by itself, it can in some instances provoke spontaneous pelvic pain mostly accompanied by deep dyspareunia.
Pathologists find chronic cervicitis in many, if not most, hysterectomy specimens, but the majority of the patients operated on have hardly any symptoms related to the cervicitis, except perhaps leukorrhea. There are, however, a few women who right after a delivery start complaining of lower abdominal pain, with or without low backache, and deep dyspareunia and who on gynecologic examination present a more or less severely torn cervix, one or two sensitive and firm uterosacral ligaments, and agglutinated leukocytes in the cervical mucus. In the absence of a history or of clinical findings suggesting the presence of endometriosis, it is reasonable to suppose that this situation is due to a chronic cellulitis, a posterior parametritis (Jeffcoate 1975), a pelvic lymphangitis (Novak et al. 1975), or "a tracking back" of the cervical infection along the sacrouterine ligaments (McClure Browne). The diagnosis "posterior parametritis due a chronic cervicitis" is all the more plausible if the spontaneous and the provoked pain disappear after treatment with antibiotics, e. g., 2 g of amoxicilline daily for 7 days, and the use of hot sitz baths or hot vaginal douches. Whenever cervical ectropion or erosion is present, it is indicated to treat the infectious process by antibiotics and to take a cervical and a vaginal smear to detect any dysplastic or malignant changes at the endoexocervical epithelial junction. If the cytologic examination is negative, it may be useful to treat the erosion by superficial electrocautery and the ectropion either by electrocautery or by trachelorrhaphy.
Once in a while, a patient with severe trichomonas vaginitis will complain of pelvic pain, and vaginal examination will reveal tenderness of the vaginal walls and of the pericervical tissues. One wonders whether, in these cases, the lower

abdominal pain may not also be due to a parametrial extension of an infectious process originating in the superficial erosions, which may be found in the vaginal fornices; this suspicion will be corroborated if the spontaneous pain disappears after adequate treatment of the vaginitis.

12.2 Chronic Salpingo-Oophoritis

The term "chronic salpingo-oophoritis" here denotes, on the one hand, tuberculous salpingitis, and on the other, the sequelae of acute PID when all clinical signs of inflammation, such as fever, leukocytosis, and elevated blood sedimentation rate, have subsided. As long as any of these signs subsists, the condition is called subacute.

Acute PID may eventuate in complete cure or may leave sequelae, such as partly deciliated and adherent folds of the tubal mucosa, a hydrosalpinx, or a tuboovarian cyst. These lesions are generally accompanied by peritubal and periovarian adhesions, but acute PID may also give rise to a subacute condition due to a pyosalpinx, an ovarian abscess, or a tubo-ovarian abscess. In other instances, a pyosalpinx or a tubo-ovarian abcess may be the end point of several episodes of recurrent salpingitis.

12.2.1 Tuberculous Salpingitis

12.2.1.1 Incidence

Genital tuberculosis used to be rather common in Western Europe until some 20–30 years ago, but at present it is becoming rare thanks to the gradual disappearance of pulmonary tuberculosis. It is wellknown indeed that in the great majority of cases, the genital – which almost always starts as a tubal localization – is secondary to a pulmonary infection. There are still many regions, including India and South-America, in which genital tuberculosis remains a problem, especially among infertility cases.

12.2.1.2 Clinical Symptoms and Signs

Table 8 shows the most frequent symptoms of genital tuberculosis according to Schaefer (1976). These symptom frequencies surely pertain to a group of patients who differ from those seen in Western Europe during the last decades;

Table 8. Symptoms of female genital tuberculosis (Schaefer 1976)

Sterility	45%–55%
Pelvic pain	c. 50%
Poor general condition	26%
Menstrual disturbances	20%
Vaginal discharge	4%

Schaefer's series must comprise a good deal of *active advanced* cases. Schockaert and Ferin (1945) and Sharman (1952) found genital tuberculosis in approximately 5%–10% of their infertility cases. Most of these patients had no symptoms, vaginal examination was mostly negative, and the tuberculous lesions were found in endometrial biopsies taken during the premenstrual phase to evaluate the luteal function. The absence of symptoms and the negative clinical examination made it possible to classify these cases as *silent or minimal* genital tuberculosis (Schaefer 1970, 1976).

In the active or advanced forms, there are general symptoms and signs of the tuberculous process; meno- or metrorrhagia and pelvic pain may be present. On pelvic examination, a fixed retroversion with palpable tubo-ovarian masses may be found. In this context, the diagnosis of genital tuberculosis becomes probable if there is no history of an ascending gonorrheal or septic infection or of a "descending" infection of the genital tract.

Pain is found only in advanced cases. Sutherland (1967) found abdominal pain in 102 of 483 patients and Schaefer (1976) in up to 50% of his cases. Several factors may explain the pain. Dyspareunia may be due to a fixed retroversion or to adherent adnexal masses. Spontaneous pain and dysmenorrhea may have their origin in a pyo- or hydrosalpinx or in a tuberculous pelviperitonitis originating in the infected tubes.

12.2.1.3 Diagnosis

Only 30% (Rozin 1975) to 50% (Schaefer 1976) of the patients have a history of *extragenital tuberculosis.* Approximately 50% of Schaefer's patients had had tuberculous pleurisy, peritonitis, or erythema nodosum or renal, osseous, or pulmonary tuberculosis.

A positive *tuberculin test* does not indicate the site of the infection; a negative tuberculin test proves with near certainty that the patient has no tuberculosis. Infection of the genital tract can be proved by the presence of tuberculous lesions in an *endometrial biopsy* or in curettings obtained preferably during the premenstrual phase of the cycle. Part of the biopsy specimen may also be innoculated in a guinea pig or cultured in *Petragnani's or Loewenstein's medium.* If these examinations are negative, repeated cultures of menstrual blood may be made. Diagnosing tuberculosis by culture has the additional advantage of allowing the determination of drug sensitivity.

Laparoscopy will reveal the presence of tuberculous lesions only infrequently and may be dangerous in the presence of tuberculous peritonitis. Due to the danger of secondary infection, hysterosalpingography should only be resorted to when the other diagnostic aids have proved negative.

12.2.1.4 Treatment

Treatment will essentially be medical, with rifamycin, isoniazid, and ethambutol, as in pulmonary tuberculosis. Drug treatment should last for a minimum of 2 years. Surgery is only indicated if the pelvic masses persist or increase, if endometrial tuberculosis persists, and if pain or other pelvic symptoms do not disappear under drug therapy.

12.2.2 Sequelae of Acute PID or "Chronic Salpingo-Oophoritis"

It is difficult to evaluate the incidence of sequelae of acute PID by clinical examination because the frequency of the acute form varies from one region to another, because the diagnosis of acute PID is not as easy as it used to be thought (Jacobson 1970), and because a reliable diagnosis would in many cases entail hysterosalpingography or laparoscopy, whereas in fact only selected groups of patients undergo these explorations. Having many years of experience with laparoscopy in the exploration of chronic pelvic pain, we are convinced that doctors tend to made the diagnosis of "chronic salpingo-oophoritis" far too frequently.

12.2.2.1 Diagnosis and Differential Diagnosis

When all signs of active inflammation have subsided in a case of acute PID, the patient may continue to complain of lower abdominal pain with premenstrual or menstrual exacerbation. In these circumstances, her symptoms are most probably due to sequelae of acute PID. They may also include dyspareunia, infertility, anomalies of the menstrual cycle, such as prolonged menstruation, shorter intervals, and sometimes signs of anovulation or of corpus luteum insufficiency. Pelvic examination may reveal enlarged and fixed adnexa, a fixed retroversion, or a sensitive posterior parametrium.

Jacobson (1970) proved by laparoscopy the presence of acute salpingitis in a series of 623 patients. This investigation constituted confirmation of a prior clinical diagnosis of acute PID in 532 cases (85%), but in the remaining 91 cases (15%), no such clinical diagnosis had previously been made. Sequelae of acute salpingitis may thus be encountered without a clinical history of an acute episode. Therefore, if the diagnosis is in doubt and if a trial of medical treatment has remained unsuccessful, laparoscopy is indicated.

The differential diagnosis between sequelae of acute PID and *„chronic appendicitis"* should not be difficult. A diagnosis of primary chronic appendicitis should only be entertained with the greatest reluctance. According to Alvarez (1943), an adult who undergoes an appendectomy for a so-called chronic appendicitis has only 1 chance in a 100 to be cured if there has not been a history of an acute episode.

Patients with lower abdominal pain due to *endometriosis* experience an acute attack of pain only infrequently. The following symptoms and signs suggest endometriosis: late menstrual dysmenorrhea, unilateral menstrual or intermenstrual pain, pain on defecation during the menstrual period, and the presence of small sensitive nodules on the posterior aspect of the uterine isthmus or in a sacrouterine ligament. The nature of adherent sensitive adnexal masses may be ascertained by puncture through the posterior fornix; a hydrosalpinx or a serous cyst will yield serous fluid, a pyosalpinx will yield pus, and an endometriotic cyst will yield syrupy, old blood. A trial of treatment with contraceptive steroids will help eight of ten patients with pain due to endometriosis, whereas this treatment is much less effective in chronic PID. Laparoscopy will generally solve the differential diagnostic problem, but here also a puncture of an adnexal mass may be necessary.

In Chap. 15, attention will be drawn to *Crohn's disease* and *disorders of the sigmoid colon.* A young patient with intermittent or progressively worsening cramplike pains in the hypogastrium or in the right iliac fossa, with bouts of diarrhea, loss of weight, slight fever, moderate leukocytosis, and an elevated blood sedimentation rate, should have a careful roentgenologic exploration of her small intestine and cecum. Patients of 40 years or more who have pain in their left iliac fossa and who observe changes in their stools or in their bowel habits, whether or not these changes are accompanied by episodes of fever, need an exploration of their large bowel, as they may have diverticulitis, peridiverticulitis, or cancer of the sigmoid.

Pelvic cellulitis or posterior parametritis due to chronic cervicitis should not be mistaken for chronic PID, the former being localized in the lower part of the parametrium and the latter in the upper genital tract; both may, however, coexist.

In Chap. 18, the necessity of differentiating "chronic pelvic pain without obvious pathology" from sequelae of chronic PID will be stressed. This differentiation can only be done by means of laparoscopy.

12.2.2.2 Explaining the Symptoms

A fixed retroversion or sensitive adnexa bound down in the pouch of Douglas easily explain deep dyspareunia. It is frequently claimed that sequelae of PID cause dysmenorrhea; in fact, if they cause spontaneous pain at all, it is generally intermenstrual pain with a premenstrual or menstrual exacerbation and not a true dysmenorrhea. The explanation of the spontaneous pain is made difficult by the fact that chronic salpingo-oophoritis is frequently asymptomatic. Comparing the adnexal lesions observed at laparoscopy in cases with painful sequelae to painless cases does not yield an explanation as to why some have pain and others do not; furthermore, there have so far been no descriptions of histologic differences between specimens obtained from both categories.

The pain may be due to circulatory changes in the internal genitalia or to contractions in the wall of a hydrosalpinx; it may also originate in a sensitive posterior parametrium. In some cases, pain at the time of ovulation or in the premenstrual phase of the cycle may be related to periovarian adhesions that interfere either with ovulation or with the development of a corpus luteum.

It would be interesting to explore patients with and patients without pain with psychometric tests, but finding two series with strictly comparable adnexal lesions would be very difficult and the interpretation of the results would be hampered by the different underlying problems of the patients: pain on the one hand and sterility on the other.

Damage to the tubal mucosa or the presence of a hydrosalpinx or of peritubal or periovarian adhesions are factors of infertility. In some cases with a shortened cycle, exploration of the luteal function by measuring the basal body temperature, by endometrial biopsy, and by determining plasma progesterone concentrations will reveal a shortened luteal phase.

12.2.2.3 Treatment

Treatment depends on what the main problem of the patient is. A search should of course be made for the cause of the infection: is it gonorrhea, an ascending septic infection, or a "descending" septic infection due to an appendicitis, to Crohn's disease, or to peridiverticulitis?
When the sequelae of PID cause infertility, some form of plastic operation will be indicated, although the prognosis is not very bright, especially when the tubal mucosa has been extensively damaged.
If the main complaint is chronic pain, anti-inflammatory drugs and local heat, either by hot vaginal douches, sitz baths, or diathermy may be tried. Surgery, even conservative surgery, should not be too easily resorted to. Conservative surgery may be indicated for a fixed retroversion causing deep dyspareunia or for gross enlargement of an adnexum. When the patient is no longer desirous of pregnancy and medical treatment does not help her, total hysterectomy with bilateral salpingo-oophorectomy is indicated. Preservation or removal of one or both ovaries will depend on their condition as evaluated during operation and on the age of the patient.

12.2.3 Subacute and Recurrent Salpingo-Oophoritis

Although acute PID and its complications are outside the scope of this text, it is worthwile to draw attention to some subacute and recurrent conditions that may create problems lasting for several weeks or months.

12.2.3.1 Pathogenetic Mechanisms

The widespread and early use of antibiotics in acute PID has reduced the frequency of pelvic peritonitis and abscess of the pouch of Douglas. On the other hand, the use of contraceptive pills and of intrauterine contraceptive devices seems to have significantly increased the danger of upper genital tract infections.
Observations by Fiumara (1971, cited by Ledger et al. 1974) show that the risk of extension of infection to the upper genital tract after exposure to gonorrhea is definitely higher in women who are taking contraceptive pills than in nonusers of the pill.
Several studies (Eschenbach 1976; Tatum 1977; Cates and Ory 1979) have shown that the incidence of upper genital tract infection is approximately four times greater in women wearing IUDs than in comparable socioeconomic groups of patients not wearing IUDs. Whereas acute PID is commonly bilateral,

several cases have been published of unilateral ovarian abscesses in IUD users.
Furthermore, there are reasons to assume that an episode of PID predisposes to a recurrence of the infection, which will then usually have a nongonococcal etiology and, indeed, will frequently be polymicrobial with a mixture of aerobic and anaerobic bacteria (Eschenbach 1976). A long-lasting subacute pelvic inflammatory process may be initiated by the propagation of a periappendicular infection, by an intestinal fistula due to Crohn's disease, or by peridiverticulitis of the sigmoid. These descending pathways of infection and the above-mentioned recurrent episodes of ascending infection are likely to lead either to a uni- or bilateral pyosalpinx or to an ovarian or a tubo-ovarian abscess, frequently combined with an abscess of the pouch of Douglas.

12.2.3.2 Diagnosis

These severe inflammatory conditions of the pelvic organs give rise to intense pain over the lower abdomen, nausea, vomiting, and abdominal distension due to paralytic ileus. The pulse rate is elevated, and the temperature is high with spikes. Palpation of the lower abdomen is exquisitely tender and there is muscle spasm. On gynecologic examination, the entire pelvis is exceedingly sensitive, and enlarged adnexal masses are felt next to the uterus. There is frequently a retroversion except when the pouch of Douglas is occupied by swollen and adherent adnexa and by an inflammatory exudate. The white blood count reaches 20000 or more, and the blood sedimentation rate is greatly accelerated.

12.2.3.3 Treatment

Treatment is medical in the acute phase, but surgical intervention may be urgently needed when there are signs of generalized peritonitis. Besides ensuring sufficient rehydration and maintaining the ionic equilibrium, it is important to provide, parenterally, an antibiotic "cover" for the pathogens most commonly found in these circumstances. Useful combinations are ampicillin plus gentamicin, penicillin plus kanamycin, or clindamycin plus gentamicin (Mead and Gump 1976; Ledger et al. 1974). This drug regimen should be continued until at least 5 days after disappearance of the fever.
When the patient fails to respond to optimal dosages of this drug therapy, reevaluation of the situation should be done to find out whether the initial diagnosis was correct or whether a complication has developed, e. g., extensive necrosis of an organ, pelvic thrombophlebitis, ovarian abscess, abscess of the pouch of Douglas, or drug fever.
An abscess of the pouch of Douglas should be drained by a posterior colpotomy. When this operation is not followed by cure and the abscess forms again, there is probably an underlying cause, e. g., an ovarian abscess that generally does not disappear after vaginal drainage or a pelvic inflammatory process initiated by Crohn's disease that is likely to subsist or recur as long as the primary condition has not been cured.

When the symptoms and signs of the disease persist for several weeks or recur intermittently, surgical exploration is indicated. The extent of the surgery will be determined by the age and the aspirations of thc paticnt and thc dcgrcc of damage suffered by the tubes or ovaries.

References

Alvarez W (1943) Nervousness, indigestion and pain. Hoeber, New York

Cates W, Ory HW (1979) I. U. D. complications: infection, death and ectopic pregnancy. In: Moghissi KS (ed) Controversies in contraception. Williams & Wilkins, Baltimore, pp 187–201

Eschenbach DA (1976) Acute pelvic inflammatory disease: strategy, risk factors and pathogenesis. Clin Obstet Gynecol 19:147–169

Jacobson L (1970) The value of visual diagnosis in acute pelvic inflammatory disease. Ned Tijdschr Verloskd 70:272–285

Jeffcoate N (1975) Principles of gynaecology, 4th edn. Butterworths, London

Ledger WJ (1975) Inflammations in infertility. In: Behrman SJ, Kistner RW (eds) Progress in infertility, 2nd edn. Little Brown, Boston, pp 207–221

Ledger WJ, Kriewall TJ, Sweet RL, Fakety F Jr (1974) The use of parenteral clindamycin in the treatment of obstetric-gynecologic patients with severe infections. A comparison of a clindamycin-kanamycin combination with penicillin-kanamycin. Obstet Gynecol 43:490–497

McClure Browne JC (1973) Postgraduate obstetrics and gynaecology. Butterworths, London

Mead PB, Gump DW (1976) Antibiotic therapy in obstetrics and gynecology. Clin Obstet Gynecol 19:109–129

Novak E, Jones JS, Jones HW (1975) Novak's textbook of gynecology, 9th edn. Williams & Wilkins, Baltimore

Rozin S (1975) Genital tuberculosis. In:Behrman SJ, Kistner RW (eds) Progress in infertility, 2nd edn. Little Brown, Boston, pp 189–206

Schaefer G (1970) Tuberculosis of the female genital tract. Clin Obstet Gynecol 13:965–998

Schaefer G (1976) Female genital tuberculosis. Clin Obstet Gynecol 19:223–239

Schockaert JA, Ferin J (1945) De endometriumbiopsie als diagnostisch hulpmiddel bij de tuberculose van de inwendige genitalia. Verh Vlaam Akad Genesk Belg 4/5: 151–166

Sharman A (1952) Endometrial tuberculosis in sterility. Fertil Steril 3:144–166

Sutherland AM (1967) Genital tuberculosis in women. Bull Sloane Hosp Women NY 13:127–141

Tatum JR (1977) Clinical aspects of intrauterine contraception: circumspection 1976. Fertil Steril 28:3–28

13 Ovarian Pain

Pain of ovarian origin is by far not as common as many doctors tend to believe. Extensive structural changes of the ovaries, such as those occurring during the menstrual cycle or during the development of ovarian cysts or tumors, mostly remain painless. The present chapter intends to give a brief survey of the conditions that may cause chronic or recurrent ovarian pain.

13.1 Ovarian Cysts

Ovarian cysts may be either functional or neoplastic, the latter being either benign or malignant. Functional cysts may be derived from a nonluteinized follicle or may be lutein cysts.

13.1.1 Follicle Cysts

Some follicle cysts are rather small, with a diameter of approximately 2.5 cm; others acquire a size of up to 8 or 10 cm in diameter. Many follicle cysts are asymptomatic and are simply incidental findings. Some are symptomatic in the sense that they may cause pelvic discomfort or heaviness; others give rise to menstrual irregularities, e. g., a delayed period or metrorrhagia, which may or may not be accompanied by pain. Such cysts mostly disappear spontaneously within a few weeks and should therefore initially be left alone. However, the patient should be examined every 3–4 weeks, and if a cyst has not disappeared within 8 weeks, it is probably neoplastic. A cystectomy or salpingo-oophorectomy is then indicated if it has characteristics of a benign growth.

When a follicle cyst manifests itself by signs of estrogen impregnation and a prolonged menstrual interval, it is indicated to prescribe a 5- or 7-day course of a progestogen to obtain an artificial menstruation and, at the same time, to prevent metrorrhagia. However, if the cyst has already caused a metrorrhagia, a short course of a progestogen will likewise be followed by a withdrawal bleeding, after which the metrorrhagia will stop.

The Stein-Leventhal or polycystic ovary syndrome should only be mentioned in this context to stress the fact that it is almost never accompanied by pain.

13.1.2 Lutein Cysts

Among the lutein cysts, a distinction has to be made between those occurring in nonpregnant women and those found during normal or abnormal pregnancy.

Some corpora lutea are cystic. It is rare for them to give rise to symptoms, unless they attain a size of several centimeters; they are then called corpus lutein cysts.

Corpus lutein cysts are usually sequelae of a corpus luteum hematoma. They may provoke unilateral pain and will raise the possibility of an ectopic preg-

nancy, especially when they are complicated by intraperitoneal hemorrhage. Differential diagnosis will be possible by means of laparoscopy.
Besides unilateral pain, a corpus luteum cyst may also result in menstrual delay. This situation raises the problem of an early pregnancy, either intra- or extrauterine. Much rarer is a persisting corpus luteum in a nonpregnant patient (Halban's syndrome).
Differentiation between these three possibilities – an early pregnancy with a corpus luteum cyst, an ectopic pregnancy, or the uncommon Halban's syndrome – will necessitate a pregnancy test and sometimes laparoscopy.
A corpus luteum cyst in early pregnancy will disappear spontaneously after a few weeks, as will also a cystic, persisting corpus luteum of Halban's syndrome. Enucleating a corpus luteum cyst in early pregnancy is a mistake, as it will jeopardize the pregnancy; indeed, this operation frequently results in an abortion.
A cystic corpus luteum or a corpus luteum cyst with or without unilateral pain may be found in some infertility cases. The luteinized unruptured follicle syndrome may indeed go together with a corpus luteum cyst. In these cases, absence of ovulation may moreover be complicated by a corpus luteum insufficiency, as shown by low 17 OH-progesterone and low plasma progesterone concentrations during the secretory phase (Abeille et al. 1978).
The *ovarian hyperstimulation syndrome,* which may be seen after induction of ovulation by means of human gonadotropins, is characterized by the presence of a variable number of corpora lutea and follicles and by edema of the ovarian stroma. In the severe grades of the syndrome, there may be lower abdominal pain. The ovaries are strikingly enlarged and tender on palpation. Treatment is conservative except in the rare cases in which there is intraperitoneal hemorrhage (Lunenfeld et al. 1969; Schenker and Weinstein 1978).
The *theca lutein cysts,* which are frequently encountered in patients with trophoblastic disease, deserve no more than mere mentioning, as they are hardly ever painful, even if they are sometimes quite large.

13.1.3 Endometriotic Cysts

In Chap. 11, we have already alluded to the fact that sizable endometriotic cysts may remain painless, whereas in other patients they may give rise to severe dysmenorrhea or continuous pain. In some cases, it seems as if the pain is conditioned by a rapid accumulation of menstrual blood and by a steep rise in intracystic pressure, but in many cases it is at present impossible to explain the mechanism of the pain or the reasons for the painlessness.

13.1.4 "Sclerocystic Ovaritis"

The terms "sclerocystic ovaritis" and more recently "painful ovarian dystrophy" have been used in the French literature to describe a syndrome with uni- or bilateral iliac fossa pain, irregular menstrual cycles, and one or two tender enlarged ovaries on palpation (Robert et al. 1974). The symptomatology of this syndrome is vague, and the findings on clinical examination vary from one case to another. The syndrome is virtually unknown in the Anglo-Saxon literature. According to Dubreuil (1947), "the sclerosis found by some pathologists in sclerocystic ovaries are normal, physiological, but temporary phenomena which become more pronounced with age but do not interfere with normal ovarian function." The points to remember are that the symptoms are generally found in neurotic patients or women with psychological problems, that removal or wedge resection of one ovary frequently leads to a recurrence of the symptoms on the other side, and that the symptoms will frequently abate under cyclic estro-progestogens.

13.1.5 Recurrent Functional Ovarian Cysts

Recently, a syndrome characterized by recurrent functional ovarian cysts in young women was described by Stone and Swartz (1979). This condition presents some analogy with the above-mentioned "painful ovarian dystrophy." They observed four patients with persistent recurrence of painful functional cysts accompanied by elevated plasma estradiol levels in three of the four in whom blood studies were done. In each of these patients, a wedge resection had been performed on the occasion of the first or the second of the painful episodes. In each patient, the mass disappeared, and recurrence could temporarily be prevented by ovarian suppression with oral contraceptives. The authors state that this syndrome may be more prevalent than a review of the literature leads one to believe. Indeed, most gynecologists have seen patients still complaining of iliac fossa pain after one or two cystectomies performed on the same ovary or after bilateral wedge resection. Surgical treatment is therefore rarely indicated in any patient who seems to harbor a functional ovarian cyst. When laparoscopy has to be performed because the diagnosis remains in doubt, it is preferable to puncture the cyst, to aspirate its contents, and to submit them to a cytologist to exclude any suspicion of malignancy (Mintz and de Brux 1974; Erb 1976). There is a great chance that the painful episode will be over.

13.2 Ovarian Remnant Syndrome

Many gynecologists have also had to deal with the ovarian remnant syndrome (Shemwell and Weed 1970). It may occur in a patient who has undergone a bilateral oophorectomy with a total abdominal hysterectomy and who has pain with or without a palpable mass or who has a palpable cystic tumor without any symptoms. The ovarian remnant syndrome may be seen when a bilateral oophorectomy has been performed in conditions that make it difficult for the surgeon to be sure that all ovarian tissue is removed e. g., when the ovaries are embedded in endometriotic scar tissue or are surrounded by dense adhesions.

For reasons that are easily understood, laparoscopy will not be very useful to diagnose this syndrome. An ovarian remnant will be suspected when the patient has evidence of estrogen secretion that still persists after a short course of corticoids to suppress adrenal androstenedione secretion. Treatment will consist in meticulous excision of the residual ovarian tissue after identification, careful dissection, and lateral displacement of the ureters (Symmonds and Pettit 1979).

13.3 Residual Ovary Syndrome

In a small percentage (approximately 3%) of all cases in which the ovaries have been left in situ at the time of hysterectomy, the patient later complains of chronic lower abdominal pain with or without dyspareunia.

Pelvic examination reveals an enlarged ovary or a unilateral pelvic mass. This condition has been called "the residual ovary syndrome" (Grogan 1967; Christ and Lotze 1975). At operation, pelvic adhesions and "perioophoritis" are frequently found. When the ovary is removed, "multiple cystic atretic and/or hemorrhagic follicles surrounded by varying degrees of peri-oophoritis are the usual histological patterns of the residual ovaries" (Grogan 1967). When only an enlarged or cystic ovary is found, it is preferable to try cyclic estroprogestogens and not to resort too easily to surgery. However, if there is a persisting pelvic mass, which might be an ovarian tumor, surgical removal is indicated.

According to the experience of Ranney and Aba-Ghazahel (1977) and Funt et al. (1977), the incidence of subsequent operations after a total nonradical hysterectomy is about 1%, which is even lower than the figure cited above. Both groups of authors therefore make a plea for the retention of normal-looking ovaries at the time of abdominal hysterectomy in the premenopausal patient; Ranney rightly insists on leaving the ovaries at the lateral end of the suture of the visceral peritoneum near the pelvic wall to prevent deep dyspareunia.

13.4 Chronic Oophoritis and Perioophoritis

Although many doctors believe chronic oophoritis to be a frequent cause of iliac fossa pain, it should be emphasized that this is only rarely the case. In chronic pelvic inflammatory disease, the ovaries are much less frequently involved than the tubes. On the other hand, "chronic perioophoritis" in the form of adhesions around one or both ovaries is a rather common sequel of acute PID. Although the ovaries may be buried under adhesions without causing pelvic pain, it is probable that dense adhesions contribute to pelvic discomfort or pain, most pronounced in the premenstrual phase in some patients. The treatment will be similar to that of sequelae of acute PID; in patients with premenstrual pain, the ovarian function may be inhibited by contraceptive steroids.

13.5 Ovarian Dyspareunia

The various causes of ovarian dyspareunia are described in Chap. 14.

13.6 Ovarian Tumors

Benign tumors of the ovary are painless unless torsion occurs or unless there is a sudden increase in the intracystic or intratumoral pressure owing to hemorrhage. The same is true for malignant tumors; they may, however, provoke pain indirectly when extracapsular growth interferes with the function of an adjacent organ.

13.7 Some Rare Causes of Ovarian Pain

We once observed a painful swelling of a residual ovary in a patient who was receiving anticoagulants. The pain was most probably due to bleeding in a follicle or corpus luteum cyst, as a great amount of blood was easily aspirated through the vaginal vault from the enlarged and fixed ovary.
About ten cases of massive unilateral edema of the ovary have been described in the literature. Most were observed in young girls. Edema and pain result from impairment of the ovarian circulation following torsion or partial torsion of the ovarian pedicle. Torsion with complete interruption of the ovarian circulation causes necrosis, but an incomplete interruption may cause edema and enlargement of the ovary, which may attain a diameter of 10–15 cm. In all cases reported, a unilateral oophorectomy was performed, but Teglbjaerg and Vetner (1977) wonder whether it would not be preferable to preserve the ovary after detorsion. Conservative surgery might, however, be hazardous as it could be complicated by postoperative embolism. Moreover, torsion of an adnexum occurs mostly, although not always, when the ovary is the seat of a tumor (Ed. Obstet Gynecol Surv 1978).
Although one hesitates to put it in writing, there seem to be cases of "painful ovary" in which no growth or microscopic evidence of disease is found, but these are exceedingly rare. This author saw only two examples in 35 years. There was a constant iliac fossa pain with fluctuations in its intensity. No explanation of the pain could be found, except that on palpation the ovary was painful and that on different occasions palpation reproduced the spontaneous pain. As no other treatment had helped the patient, the tender ovary was removed and the pain disappeared. Atlee (1966), who was very sceptical about many pain causes and syndromes described in the literature, "grudgingly" admitted that he had relieved a few patients by surgically removing such a normal-looking but painful ovary. We have to agree with Jeffcoate (1975) who states that there is no such thing as ovarian dysmenorrhea. "Ovarian dysmenorrhea" has been described by some gynecologists (Browne 1949; Atlee 1966) in cases were the ovaries appeared normal but were tender on examination.

References

Abeille JP, Moing MH, Legros R, Scholler R, Castanier M, Nahoul K (1978) Le corps jaune kystique. Un aspect celioscopique particulier de la pathologie fonctionelle ovarienne. Confrontation laparo-biologique. Rev Fr Gynecol 73:19–27

Atlee HB (1966) Acute and chronic iliac pain in women. A problem of diagnosis, 2nd edn. Thomas, Springfield III, p 123
Browne OD (1949) A survey of 113 cases of primary dysmenorrhea treated by neurectomy. Am J Obstet Gynecol 57:1053–1068
Christ JL, Lotze EC (1975) The residual ovary syndrome. Obstet Gynecol 46:551–566
Dubreuil G (1947) L'ovaire féminin envisagé à la lueur de récentes acquisitions morphologiques et histopathologiques. In: Cotte G (ed) L'ovulation et ses troubles. L'Expansion Scientifique Française, Paris, pp 5–43
Erb H (1976) Diagnostisches und therapeutisches Vorgehen bei kleinen Ovarialtumoren. Schweiz Rundsch Med (Praxis) 65:167–171
Funt MI, Benigno BB, Thompson JD (1977) The residual adnexa. Asset or liability. Am J Obstet Gynecol 129:251–254
Grogan RH (1967) Reappraisal of residual ovaries. Am J Obstet Gynecol 97:124–129
Jeffcoate N (1975) Principles of gynaecology, 4th edn. Butterworths, London
Lunenfeld B, Insler V, Rabau E (1969) Induction de l'ovulation par les gonadotrophines. In: Moricard R, Ferin J (eds) L'ovulation. Masson, Paris, pp 291–340
Mintz M, de Brux J (1974) La ponction percelioscopique et la cytologie de 347 kystes intrapelviens. Gynecologie 25:63–75
Ranney B, Abu-Ghazaleh S (1977) The future function and fortune of ovarian tissue which is retained in situ during hysterectomy. Am J Obstet Gynecol 128:626–634
Robert HG, Palmer R, Boury-Heyler C, Cohen J (1974) Précis de gynécologie. Masson, Paris
Schenker J, Weinstein D (1978) Ovarian hyperstimulation syndrome: a current survey. Fertil Steril 30:255–268
Shemwell RE, Weed JC (1970) Ovarian remnant syndrome. Obstet Gynecol 36:299–303
Stone SC, Swartz WJ (1979) A syndrome characterized by recurrent symptomatic functional ovarian cysts in young women. Am J Obstet Gynecol 134:310–314
Symmonds RE, Pettit PDN (1979) Ovarian remnant syndrome. Am J Obstet Gynecol 54:174–177
Teglbjaerg PS, Vetner M (1977) A case of massive unilateral oedema of the ovary simulating tumour. Acta Obstet Gynecol Scand 56:157–159

14 Dyspareunia

Dyspareunia, or pain during or after intercourse, is a common complaint in gynecologic practice. It is usually one of several symptoms in patients consulting for chronic pelvic pain, but nowadays dyspareunia is no longer an infrequent complaint, even if some patients will admit this important form of sexual dysfunction only after a detailed history. In light of the modern emphasis of individuals as well as of married people on sexual gratification and its unquestionable importance in fomenting and maintaining mutual understanding in marriage, this complaint should never be taken lightly.

14.1 Varieties of Dyspareunia

Depending on the initiating circumstances, the localization, or the predominant cause, several varieties of dyspareunia may be distinguished. Dyspareunia is called *primary* when it has existed ever since the first intercourse and *secondary* when it appeared at some later date. It is *superficial* if the pain is localized at the level of the vulva and the vagina introitus, *vaginal* if experienced at the level of the vaginal walls, and *deep* if deep thrusting of the penis hurts tender organs or tissues in the depth of the vagina and pelvis.

There is some discussion as to the relative frequency of *organic* and *psychogenic* dyspareunia. The majority of the cases seem to have organic origins, but as psychosomatic interactions are liable to intervene in every case of dyspareunia, attempts should be made to find out for each patient individually which factor or factors are preponderant in the pathogenesis of the symptom.

We will mainly review the most frequent organic causes and will briefly consider the psychological issues and the psychophysiologic mechanisms that may provoke, complicate, or entertain dyspareunia.

An organic cause can usually be identified easily, either because the patient will clearly describe the localization of her pain or because the doctor can reproduce the pain on gynecologic examination.

14.2 Superficial Dyspareunia

If superficial dyspareunia is experienced when a girl or a woman starts having sexual relations, it may be due to a *rigid hymen* or to *irritated or bruised remnants of the hymen.* A rigid hymen may be found in a woman who began having intercourse only in her 30s or 40s. Usually, however, it is not so much the hymen that is rigid; frequently there will be an underlying problem, such as emotional unpreparedness for coitus or fear of coitus or of pain. The pain complaint may be associated with a more or less intense contraction of the sphincter vaginae (m. bulbocavernosus) and sometimes of the deeper muscles of the perineum, especially the levator ani muscle, and the adductors of the thigh; we are then dealing not only with dyspareunia but with vaginismus. In these cases, treatment should start by psychotherapy. If there are no concomitant contractions of the perineal muscles, a rigid or tender hymen can best be treated by self-dilation of the hymen with progressively larger dilators, which are well-lubricated with a nonirritating lubricant. In a collaborating patient, a hymenotomy can be performed under local anesthesia. A dilation of the hymen can also be performed under anesthesia with a small Cusco speculum. If there are irritated or bruised remnants of the hymen, sexual rest should be prescribed for some time and, before intercourse is resumed, progressive self-dilation is advisable.

When there is a *hymen septum,* with two orifices separated by a median septum, this septum should be divided.

When *a cyst of a Bartholin's gland or chronic bartholinitis* cause dyspareunia, the cyst should be marsupialized; a swollen gland that remains tender after treatment with local heat should be excised.

Among the urologic causes should be mentioned: an abscess of a Skene's gland, prolapse of urethral mucosa, the "urethral syndrome," and diverticula of the urethra.

A tender *abscess of a Skene's gland* should be incised and drained. When there is *prolapse of the urethral mucosa,* the redundant mucosa should be resected. The so-called *urethral syndrome* is characterized by dysuria, frequency of micturition, suprapubic discomfort, and occasionally by dyspareunia; there is often a history of hematuria, which may have been noticed on the toilet paper after voiding. In many instances, the "urethral syndrome" appears to be the result of pathogenic organisms that the patient harbors in the vagina, vulval introitus, and urethra (Jacobo 1978). The best treatment seems to consist in the oral administration of trimethroprim sulfamethoxazole, which reduces the number of pathogenic organisms in the vaginal and urethral flora.

A *diverticulum of the urethra* is not seen frequently but may sometimes go unrecognized. Milking the urethra will yield a small spurt of cloudy urine and will help in localizing the diverticulum. After careful localization by means of a double-balloon Davis-Te Linde catheter, the diverticulum should be excised transvaginally, and the urethral mucosa, the bed of the diverticulum, and the vaginal mucosa should be closed in three layers.

14.2.1 Tender Episiotomy Scars

Dyspareunia is seen rather frequently right after a delivery; it is then usually due to an excessively tight repair of the perineum, which may remain tender for several weeks. The condition is treated by hot sitz baths and by applying a lubricating jelly; vaginal dilators may also be useful. Surgical correction is sometimes indicated when a tender episiotomy scar is the result either of an asymmetric suture or of the breakdown of an episiotomy wound by infection. Tenderness of an episiotomy or a postoperative scar may sometimes be due to a neuroma, but when the scar is well-reconstructed from an anatomic viewpoint, it should be revised only rarely. It may be infiltrated with depot cortisol dissolved in a local anesthetic, and if this does not help, the scar should be stretched by progressive self-dilation of the vulva and the vaginal wall.

14.2.2 Posterior Repair Scars

Jeffcoate (1959) and Francis and Jeffcoate (1961) drew attention to the frequency of overzealous posterior repairs as a cause of dyspareunia. In a series of patients operated on by Jeffcoate, they found that 20% of the women who had had repair operations for prolapse subsequently suffered from apareunia or dyspareunia owing to narrowness of the vagina. This was partly due to a senile atrophy that supervened after the operation and partly because a colpoperineorrhaphy had been combined with the anterior repair. The authors therefore feel that posterior repair should be avoided in all cases except when it is clearly indicated, e. g., by the presence of a symptom causing rectocele. The amount of vaginal mucosa that is removed should be strictly limited, given that the vagina will become narrower with the development of senile atrophy. Francis and Jeffcoate also state that the patient should be examined some 2–3 weeks after surgery to separate any loose adhesions that may have formed after the operation and a second time after 6 weeks. If the scars are well-healed after 6 weeks, the patient need not hesitate to resume intercourse. Having found a high frequency of apareunia and dyspareunia in a series of patients of his own, Simmons (1963) considers it advisable to abandon the excision of a triangle of vaginal mucosa and to stop making an inverted T incision at the perineal hedge at the beginning of a posterior repair. He recommends performing a small median episiotomy, without excision of perineal skin, followed by the resection of redundant vaginal mucosa to expose the levator ani and perineal muscles, which should be approximated under the mucosa and the skin. As Simmons showed in another series of patients, this technique does not result in a thin and tender "skin bridge," which so frequently causes dyspareunia.

14.2.3 Senile Atrophy

Narrowing of the vulval introitus may be caused by atrophy after menopause or castration or by shrinkage due to kraurosis or lichen sclerosus et atrophicus. If the dyspareunia is not cured by progressive self-dilation and the administration of estrogens in postmenopausal women, surgical dilation of the introitus may be performed. This may be done by a median incision of the fourchette, followed by undermining of the vaginal mucosa and the perineal skin and by approximating mucosa and skin with interrupted sutures disposed in a transverse direction. It may also be done by means of Z-plasty (Rankin 1973; Käser et al. 1973).

14.2.4 Perineal Endometriosis

A focus of endometriosis in an episiotomy scar is an uncommon cause of superficial dyspareunia. The lesion may be excised if it is well-localized, but more diffuse lesions that would entail the removal of a sizable part of perineal tissue or a focus that infiltrates the anal sphincter are better left alone and treated either with estroprogestogens or with the continuous administration of a progestogen, e. g., 5 mg of ethinylestrenol or 5 mg of norethisterone acetate daily for several months.

14.3 Vaginal Dyspareunia

Either organic conditions found in the vaginal wall or psychosomatic factors resulting in insufficient lubrification of the vaginal wall can cause vaginal dyspareunia (Masters and Johnson 1970; Fordney 1978). The most frequent among the *organic causes* are the cases of vaginitis.

Candida albicans vaginitis may be diagnosed on the basis of its clinical features and by finding the fungi either in a saline wet mount, a potassium hydroxide wet mount, or in a fungal culture. The treatment of this sometimes resistant disorder will not be discussed here.

Only severe cases of *Trichomonas vaginalis* vaginitis give rise to dyspareunia; the less severe forms cause only leukorrhea with or without pruritus. In severe cases, the clinical symptoms and signs are very suggestive, and the diagnosis is verified by a saline wet mount, which should be examined under the microscope immediately. Treatment will be effective only if directed at both the woman and her husband or sexual partner.

Although there is some discussion as to its pathogenicity, it must be admitted that *Hemophilus vaginalis* causes a vaginitis that has to be differentiated from *T. vaginalis* vaginitis. *H. vaginalis* vaginitis is characterized by a gray homogeneous and malodorous discharge, which may sometimes be slightly frothy. The diagnosis is established by finding many "clue cells" in a wet mount. Clue cells are epithelial cells that appear stippled or granulated due to the adherence of many *H. vaginalis* (short gram-negative) bacilli on the surface of the cell. This condition should be treated by sulfacream applied intravaginally for 10–15 days, and to prevent reinfections, the patient and her partner should receive a systemic treatment with 500 mg of ampicillin (four times daily) for 5 or 6 days (Gardner 1975).

Postmenopausal atrophy of the vagina explains many cases of dyspareunia in older patients. This atrophy is rather frequently complicated by a vaginitis (senile vaginitis). Treatment of the mucosal atrophy is by estrogens, e. g., 2–4 mg of estriol daily for 25 days/month. In cases of severe atrophy, a biphasic treatment with estrogens followed by estrogens and progestogens may be prescribed. Patients who still have their uterus should be warned that they will have artificial menstruations. When, besides the atrophy, there is also senile vaginitis, the systemic estrogen treatment should be combined with intravaginal sulfonamide cream or sulfonamide tablets daily for 10–14 days.

Tenderness of the vaginal wall may sometimes result from a *hypersensitivity* to contraceptive jellies or creams or to the lubricating coating of condoms. A medial septum of the vagina will frequently remain unnoticed, but a *transverse* septum or a *stenosis of the vagina* may cause severe dyspareunia. A transverse septum will have to be excised. A congenital or acquired stenosis of the vagina may be treated by radial incisions and digital dilation, by a longitudinal incision with transverse suture, by Z-plasty, or by the technique of Granjon (Käser et al. 1973). In all these instances, it is important to maintain the result of the surgical correction by repeated vaginal self-dilation and by resuming intercourse as soon as possible. When the *vaginal barrel* has become *too short,* e. g., after a Wertheim-Meigs operation for cervical carcinoma, vulvovaginoplasty may be performed according to the technique of Williams (1964), which uses the labia majora to lengthen the vagina (Haspels 1977). If the patient has also undergone a bilateral oophorectomy, the result of this operation will be improved by prescribing systemic estrogens.

Some *contraceptive methods* may interfere with adequate lubrication of the vagina. This may be the case with condoms that are insufficiently lubricated. Systemic progestogen injection, e. g., medroxyprogesterone acetate (depot Provera), the continuous daily ingestion of 5 mg of ethinyl-estrenol (Orgametril), or norethisterone acetate (Primolut N or R), may cause a mild state of atrophy of the vaginal mucosa; this may be corrected by the administration of small doses of estrogens (Thiery 1971).

Psychogenic Dyspareunia

Psychological factors may by themselves lead to dyspareunia (primary psychogenic dyspareunia) or may act as secondary consequences of organic disorders (secondary psychogenic dyspareunia).

According to Masters and Johnson (1970), the psychophysiologic mechanism at work here is insufficient vaginal lubrication during intercourse; this may result in burning, itching, and aching. There are many emotional issues that may be associated with *primary psychogenic dyspareunia.* They may be related to sexual behavior, e. g., fear of intercourse, the clumsy sexual technique of the partner, fear of pregnancy, temporary problems in the marital relationship, or lack of interest in, or aversion to, the husband or partner. Psychogenic dyspareunia may also be the consequence of a depressive state that may either be endogenous or may be exogenous around or after the menopause, after sterilization, or after hysterectomy. When a careful examination of the patient does not disclose an organic cause of the dyspareunia, one should enquire about psychogenic factors, which when present may be cared for either by the general practitioner or the gynecologist, but which will have to be referred to a sexual dysfunction clinic in difficult situations (Milne 1976; Fordney 1978; Craig and Milne 1978).

Many cases of organic dyspareunia are compounded by insufficient vaginal lubrication through lack of adequate sexual stimulation, which is itself due to fear of pain *(secondary psychogenic dyspareunia).* One should then try to eliminate the organic cause, but even after appropriate treatment of this condition, it may be necessary to resort to deconditioning and relearning techniques, such as vaginal self-dilation exercises (Fordney 1978).

14.4 Deep Dyspareunia

The fact that there are, in the depth of the female pelvis, several organs and tissues that may become sensitive for varying periods during the life time of a woman explains that deep dyspareunia is frequent and its pathogenesis diversified. The paracervical or parametrial tissues or ligaments may become tender as a result of an infectious process originating in the cervix *(pelvic cellulitis or parametritis).* When this condition causes deep dyspareunia, the pain may be reproduced by lifting the cervix or stretching the uterosacral ligaments. Systemic treatment with broad-spectrum antibiotics, such as amoxicillin (Clamoxyl), aims at eradicating the focus of infection, and local heat, applied either by hot sitz baths, by hot vaginal douches, or by diathermy, will activate the resorption of the inflammatory process.

In most cases of *chronic pelvic pain without abvious pathology,* the posterior parametrial tissues will be tender, and anteroposterior condensations may be found, sometimes accompanied by shortening of the posterior parametrium, although there are no signs of an infectious process. This pathologic entity will only be diagnosed when there are reasons to assume that the pain has a gynecologic origin and when careful examination, including laparoscopy, has demonstrated the absence of any obvious organic cause. For the pathogenesis and the treatment of this enigmatic syndrome see Chap. 18.

Allen and Masters (1955) and Allen (1970) have described a series of patients whose chronic pelvic pain and deep dyspareunia they attributed to *traumatic lacerations of uterine support.* In a paper on chronic pelvic pain without obvious pathology (Renaer et al. 1980), the author has shown that in his practice and in that of several other European gynecologists, this condition is rarely seen.

Painful scars in one or in both vaginal fornices, resulting from a deep cervical or vaginal tear, have fortunately become rare since the abolition of difficult forceps applications in obstetric practice. Treatment of deep dyspareunia caused by this kind of scar may be very difficult and sometimes a total nonradical hysterectomy with excision of the scar tissue will have to be performed.

Pelvic endometriosis is a frequent cause of dyspareunia when its foci are localized in the uterosacral ligaments, on fixed adnexa, or when they have resulted in a fixed retroversion of the uterus. Depending on the particular circumstances of the case, treatment will be medical or surgical or combined (see Chap. 11).

Most retroverted-retroflected uteri are symptomless, but in some patients deep thrusting movements of the penis may cause pain by exerting pressure on a *tender retroflected uterus.* If the uterus is mobile, the dyspareunia may be relieved after reduction of the retroversion and insertion of a Smith or Hodge pessary; operative reduction will seldom be necessary. Operative reduction or hysterectomy will sometimes be performed when there is severe deep dyspareunia that is due to a fixed retroversion.

If the patient's pain can be reproduced by digital pressure on an *adnexum* that is *prolapsed* and *adherent* in the pouch of Douglas, resection of the adhesions or a salpingo-oophorectomy may be indicated.

By means of intrauterine radiotelemetry pressure pills, Fox et al. (1970) have shown that there is a rise in intrauterine pressure of approximately 40 cm of water during female orgasm. This may explain the rare cases in which orgasm is experienced as *uterine cramps.*

Surgical operations may cause superficial, vaginal, as well as deep dyspareunia.

Abnormal shortening of the vagina after a Wertheim-Meigs operation for cancer of the cervix has already been mentioned. The vagina may also be shortened after an anterior repair that results in obliteration of the anterior vault; this unfortunate situation can be prevented by preservation of a sufficient length of vaginal wall, whose edges should be approximated by interrupted sutures. The same holds true for the repair of the vaginal wall during a vaginal hysterectomy.

A painful vaginal vault scar causing deep dyspareunia is sometimes found after an abdominal hysterectomy. If this is due to an endometriotic lesion, it may be destroyed by electrocautery. The same treatment may be used for a painful crestlike projection from an uneven scar in the depth of the vagina. Painful spots in the vaginal vault scar after a total hysterectomy may be infiltrated with a depot corticoid dissolved in a local anesthetic. If the spontaneous pain or the dyspareunia recurs, a resection of the painful area of the scar may be tried, as it may be the site of a neuroma; however, one should first study the personality and the behavior of the patient since in this as in other cases the complaint may be a conscious or unconscious means to avoid intercourse.

When confronted with the complaint of deep dyspareunia, one may as a symptomatic treatment suggest avoiding deep vaginal penetration during coitus. This may be realized by the wife adducting and extending both thighs after penetration or by the partners adopting the lateral coital position, either vis-à-vis or a tergo. Although one would suppose these positions to be efficient in most cases, the deep dyspareunia sometimes persists. The explanation may be that the sensitive tissues or organs are still being hurt in spite of the modified coital technique. The persisting pain may also be due to the traction that the parametrial smooth muscle fibers can exercise during the "cervical elevation" of the female's excitement phase (Masters and Johnson 1966) on inelastic and tender pelvic tissues. It may, however, also result from psychological factors underlying the complaint of dyspareunia.

14.5 Psychological Factors

The syndrome of *vaginismus* has been mentioned during the discussion of superficial dyspareunia. All causes of dyspareunia can – secondarily to the pain – provoke vaginismus, thus representing a defense mechanism. However, in a large percentage of cases, vaginismus is primary, i. e., of psychogenic origin, denoting sexual inexperience, emotional unpreparedness, fear of coitus or of pain, etc. Normal organic findings, demonstration of pelvic and perineal muscle control, prescription of self-exploration with Perspex pegs ("dilators") and also digital exploration, together with psychotherapy may help the patient. Dilation of the hymen under general anesthesia or vulvotomy will rarely cure the symptom.

Primary and secondary *psychogenic dyspareunia* has been discussed in Sect. 14.3, an important psychophysiologic mechanism being insufficient vaginal lubrication during intercourse. Psychological factors underlying the complaint of deep dyspareunia have also been mentioned; deep dyspareunia can indeed function as the means, conscious or unconscious, to avoid intercourse.

So far, this review of the possible causes of dyspareunia has placed a rather strong emphasis on organic conditions. This should not blind us to the fact that in the pathogenesis of many cases of dyspareunia, psychological and organic factors blend. In some cases, psychological issues will be preponderant and in others, organic causes; however, we should be on the alert for the mixed cases so as not to disregard the complexity of the problem.

Curing an organic condition will not automatically cure the psychophysiologic consequences of the lack of sexual stimulation conditioned by the fear of pain. The same holds true when the dyspareunia has been used for a long time as an excuse to avoid intercourse. The psychotherapeutic aftercare needed may consist in simple deconditioning and reeducation exercises, but when the dyspareunia is either a cause or a consequence of problems in the partners' interpersonal relationship, it may be necessary to call upon specialized psychotherapeutic help.

References

Allen WM (1970) Chronic pelvic congestion and pelvic pain. Am J Obstet Gynecol 109:198–202
Allen WM, Masters WH (1955) Traumatic laceration of uterine support. Am J Obstet Gynecol 70:500–513
Craig GA, Milne HB (1978) Sexual dysfunction. In: MacDonald RR (ed) Scientific basis of obstetrics and gynaecology. Churchill-Livingstone, Edinborough London, pp 525–551
Fordney DS (1978) Dyspareunia and vaginismus. Clin Obstet Gynecol 21:205–221
Fox CA, Wolff HS, Baker JA (1970) Measurement of intravaginal and intrauterine pressures during human coitus by radio-telemetry. J Reprod Fertil 33:69–75
Francis WJA, Jeffcoate TNA (1961) Dyspareunia following vaginal operations. J Obstet Gynaecol Br Commonw 68:1–10
Gardner HI (1975) The vulvo-vaginitides. (New interpretations and treatment methods). In: Taymor ML, Green TH (eds) Progress in gynecology. Grune & Stratton, New York 307–338
Haspels AA (1977) Iatrogenic dyspareunia after gynaecological treatment. In: Musaph H, Haspels AA (eds) Dyspareunia. Aspects of painful coitus. Bohn Scheltema & Holkema, Utrecht, pp 74–86
Jacobo E (1978) Diseases of the urethra. In: Buchsbaum HJ, Schmidt JD (eds) Gynecologic and obstetric urology. Saunders, Philadelphia London, pp 325–346
Jeffcoate TNA (1959) Posterior colpoperineorrhaphy. Am J Obstet Gynecol 77: 490–502
Käser O, Ikle FA, Hirsch HA (1973) Atlas der gynäkologischen Operationen, 3rd edn. Thieme, Stuttgart
Masters WH, Johnson VE (1966) Human sexual response. Little Brown, Boston
Masters H, Johnson VE (1970) Human sexual inadequacy. Churchill, London
Milne HB (1976) The role of the psychiatrist. In: Milne HB, Hardy S (eds) Psychosexual problems. Crosby Lockwood Stapels, London, pp 65–87
Rankin RP (1973) The use of Z-plasty in gynecologic operations: Case reports. Am J Obstet Gynecol 117:231–232
Renaer M, Nijs P, van Assche A, Vertommen H (1980) Chronic pelvic pain without obvious pathology in women. Eur J Obstet Gynecol Reprod Biol 10/6 pp 415–463
Simmons SC (1963) Dyspareunia following repair; the "skin bridge" and its prevention. J Obstet Gynaecol Br Commonw 70:476–478
Thiery M, Buyse G, Haspels AA (1971) Anticonceptie. Stafleu, Leiden
Williams EA (1964) Congenital absence of the vagina. A simple operation for its relief. J Obstet Gynaecol Br Commonw 71:511–516

15 Acute and Chronic Lower Abdominal Pain of Enterocolic Origin

(N. C. Hightower and J. W. Roberts)

Pain of enterocolic origin is one of the most common complaints the physician encounters in his medical practice. Whereas pain due to a musculoskeletal disorder is usually so well-localized and its qualities so characteristic that an experienced orthopedist often can easily and promptly make the correct diagnosis, this is usually not the case for pain of enterocolic origin. The abdominal viscera of the gut and its appendages are relatively inaccessible to the classic methods of examinations: inspection, palpation, auscultation, and percussion. Thus, the diagnostic skills of a physician examining a patient with abdominal pain of enterocolic origin are often taxed. Fortunately, however, a skillfully taken medical history and meticulous examination of the abdomen will usually result in a diagnosis that needs confirmation in only about 75% of patients. The remaining 25% of patients may require great effort and resourcefulness on the part of the physician before a correct diagnosis can be made.

The alimentary tract has three principal functions that occur simultaneously along with the intraluminal digestive processes; these are secretion, absorption, and motility. Although secretory and absorptive disorders undoubtedly influence gastric and intestinal symptoms, the secretory and absorptive mechanisms per se do not give rise to pain. We are left then with the motor activity or a neuromuscular disorder of the gut to explain the pain of enterocolic origin.

15.1 Innervation and Visceral Sensations

Although the alimentary canal of man has an extensive extrinsic as well as intrinsic nerve supply, it is relatively insensitive to the stimuli that ordinarily produce pain (Hightower and Janowitz 1978).

15.1.1 Innervation

The gastrointestinal tract receives an abundant nerve supply via the autonomic nerves. Cerebrospinal nerves supply the lesser omentum, the mesentery, and the mesocolon as well as the parietal peritoneum. In the mesentery, the cerebrospinal nerve endings terminate about 2 cm from the gut.

The autonomic nerves are classified as sympathetic and parasympathetic; however, it is more in keeping with modern thought to consider them as cholinergic or adrenergic depending on whether they liberate acetylcholine or epinephrine-like substances at their final terminations. Thus, most parasympathetic nerves are cholinergic and most sympathetics nerves are adrenergic, but there is considerable mixing since there are many cholinergic fibers in the sympathetic nerves supplying the gut.

In addition, the gut contains within its walls elaborate plexuses of interconnecting ganglia. These ganglia consist of the myenteric plexus, situated between the circular and longitudinal layers of the smooth muscle, and the submucous plexus, situated in the submucosa.

The parasympathetic nerve supply to the gastrointestinal smooth muscle comes mainly from the vagus, which innervates the upper gastrointestinal tract, the small bowel, and the proximal portion of the colon. The parasympathetic pelvic nerves supply the distal portion of the colon, sigmoid, and rectum. The parasympathetic fibers, whether vagus or pelvic in origin, do not end directly on the smooth muscle cells but end by making synapses with cells in the enteric plexuses. Thus, they stand in relation to these plexuses as intercalated or internuncial fibers between reflex centers and not as ordinary motor nerve fibers. The function of these fibers in the central nervous system and presumably in this situation also is to increase or decrease the excitability of the reflex centers and not to initiate muscular activity directly.

The sympathetic supply to the stomach and small intestine is by way of the splanchnic nerves. The cecum, appendix, and ascending and transverse colon are supplied by nerves that arise from the superior mesenteric plexus. The distal colon, sigmoid, and the rectum are supplied by sympathetic fibers, which arise from the upper and lower divisions of the hypogastric plexus. The preganglionic sympathetic fibers end in the celiac, aortic, or the superior or inferior mesenteric ganglia. The fibers that reach the intestines therefore are postganglionic. They probably have no function related to the enteric plexuses, even though they traverse the enteric ganglia and are distributed along with the postganglionic enteric plexus fibers. It is thought that the sympathetic innervation is concerned primarily with the vasomotor activity of the numerous blood vessels in the intestines, but some go to the intestinal smooth muscle in the muscular mucosa (Kuntz 1953).

The gastrointestinal tract is capable of carrying on its major functions after all the extrinsic nerves have been severed. This automoticity may be attributed partly to local nervous mechanisms and partly to the properties of the smooth muscle itself. Probably the essentially rhythmic functions, such as gastric antral peristalsis and segmenting contractions of the small and large intestine, are dependent upon the properties of the smooth muscle and its myoelectric activity. The more highly coordinated functions, such as forward peristalsis in the small intestine and mass movements in the colon, are thought to be dependent upon the functional integrity of the myenteric plexuses. Both the neurogenic and myogenic functions are modulated through central nervous system reflexes by way of the autonomic nerves.

15.1.2 Visceral Sensations

The abdominal and thoracic viscera are insensitive to several types of stimuli, which readily arouse sensations in the skin and more superficial tissues of the body. The effects of different varieties of stimuli, such as thermal, chemical, tactile, painful stimuli, have been investigated by a large number of observers. Sensations from the digestive tract are not readily produced or appreciated. In fact, the exposed stomach or intestine can be cut, pinched, cauterized, or stitched without producing pain. How can these observations be reconciled with the well-known fact that pain is one of the most common manifestations of visceral disease? It is known that pathologic conditions, such as ulceration, inflammation, edema, or obstruction of the bowel, may result in abdominal pain or cramping that may be very severe. Most of the available evidence indicates that the normal digestive tract is insensitive, and we seldom perceive its normal functions, especially its motor activity. Conscious appreciation only results from chemical or mechanical stimulation of the diseased or inflamed portions of the gut. Deprivation of blood supply to the digestive tract also produces sensations and may be responsible for the distress associated with severe distention or

spasm. Griping or colic sensations normally experienced with diarrheal disorders vary with the rate of intestinal contractions.
The sensation of touch disappears at the lower end of the pharynx. The rectum possesses no tactile sensibility, but the anal canal is sensitive to thermal stimuli. The esophagus is sensitive to extremes of heat and cold.
Chemicals with the exception of alcohol cause no sensation whatever when introduced into the stomach or intestinal canal. The mucosa is completely insensitive to acids. Alcohol stimulates the mucosa of the esophagus and stomach and causes a sensation of warmth. Peppermint and various condiments free from alcohol arouse no sensation. The pelvic colon and rectum show a similar sensitivity to alcohol but are insensitive to other chemicals. The anal canal is extremely sensitive, especially to alcohol and glycerin, which causes a burning sensation.
It should be remembered that the whole subject of pain arising in or referred from the viscera is still controversial and not completely understood.

15.2 General Considerations of Enterocolic Pain

An evaluation of lower abdominal pain due to enterocolic origin can be most difficult. However, if a few general principles are kept in mind, one can usually arrive at a reasonably accurate estimation of the origin of the enterocolic pain.

15.2.1 Visceral Pain

The most common cause of enterocolic visceral pain is thought to be spasm or stretch of the smooth muscle that makes up the wall of the viscus. The pain receptors of the splanchnic afferent nerve fibers are the corpuscles of Pacini as well as free nerve endings in the wall of the bowel. Visceral pain is poorly localized, and depending upon its cause may vary from a burning or "gnawing," aching sensation that may be dull or sharp to that of cramping. Most often, visceral pain is felt in the midline of the abdomen. Poor localization of visceral pain may be due to the fact that the afferent fibers carrying the pain impulses are spread over a large segment of the splanchnic innervation. Another explanation is that the patient may not be able to accurately localize the visceral pain because visceral impulses rarely reach conscious levels. Thus, there is limited experience in appreciating visceral sensations. Impulses conducted over the cerebrospinal pathways are continuously reaching conscious levels and are easily recognized and well-localized. In addition, the cortical representation of visceral structures is very limited in comparison to the extensive cortical areas receiving impulses from receptors in somatic and cutaneous surfaces.
There are a number of phenomena commonly associated with visceral pain, especially if severe. These include restlessness, nausea, vomiting, pallor, and sweating. The patient will often assume various odd positions in an attempt to relieve pain. Severe visceral pain usually provokes activity, such as doubling over, writhing, or squirming in an attempt to obtain relief. Thus, the patient may

seem to be restless and in almost constant motion in an attempt to relieve the discomfort.

Like the pains of dysmenorrhea or childbirth, the pain of intestinal colic, although diffuse, seems to arise within the organ itself even when referred to a somatic structure, such as muscles or skin.

Although it was originally thought that pain could not arise in a normal viscus, it is now known that a normal viscus may give rise to pain from a disease in a distant organ through a visceral motor reflex. Thus, painful contractions of the small intestine may accompany disease of the appendix. Hurst, as early as 1911, concluded that the only adequate stimulus for visceral pain was tension (Hurst 1911). Thus, distention of a hollow viscus or spasm over a segment of the small intestine or colon can give rise to pain as a result of the stretch stimulus applied to the nerve terminals in its wall.

Although the question is by no means settled, it appears that contraction of the muscular wall of a hollow viscus, such as the intestine, does not cause pain unless the movement of the bowel results in traction upon the mesentery. Pain arises, however, if the contraction caused distention of a neighboring portion of the wall as may result when the contraction wave approaches a mechanical obstruction, a segment of bowel in spasm, or a sphincter that fails to relax. Distension of the human appendix by the injection of fluids through an appencostomy opening causes severe pain in the epigastrium or in the region of McBurney's point. When the duodenum is distended by a balloon or injection of material through a duodenal tube, pain is felt on the right side of the epigastrium. Bentley and Smithwick (1940) distended the jejunum of patients whose splanchnic nerves had been divided on one or both sides. After unilateral denervation, distention caused pain on the unoperated side only. No pain whatever was felt after bilateral splanchnic section.

15.2.2 Somatic Pain

The receptors for somatic pain are the free nerve endings of the cerebrospinal nerves supplying the mesentery and peritoneum. Somatic pain is well-localized and usually asymmetric. If severe, it may be aggravated by walking, jarring, or even riding in an automobile. The restless movements of the patient with severe visceral pain are in striking contrast to the patient suffering from severe somatic pain. With severe somatic pain, the patient does not want to be moved, remains quiet, and resists any activity.

The same thoracic segments (T6–12,) that provide the splanchnic innervation of the alimentary canal also supply cerebrospinal innervation to the anterior and lateral parietal peritoneal surfaces. Since the anterior portion of the peritoneum does not have bilateral innervation, somatic pain conducted over the cerebrospinal segments is appreciated and identified with the dermatome supplied by the cerebrospinal nerves. Thus, pain arising in the parietal peritoneum is sharp and more discrete and is felt in the abdominal wall directly over the affected structures or affected tissues. Somatic pain is associated with tenderness on abdominal palpation. Severe somatic pain, such as occurs from a perforated viscus or an intra-abdominal abscess, is usually associated with muscle guarding or marked rigidity of the rectus muscles of the abdomen.

15.2.3 Referred Pain

The term "referred" is applied whenever pain is felt at a site other than the region affected by the pathologic process. At times, the referred pain may be felt at a distance from the stimulus because involved afferent nerves derive from a distant neurosegment. The classic example is that irritation of the inferior surface of the diaphragm can cause shoulder pain.

When a viscus is diseased, pain or tenderness is frequently felt in the tissues approximately overlying it or in some part quite remote from it. For example, pain is felt in the neck or shoulder in conditions affecting the diaphragm, between the scapula in gastric or pancreatic disease, and in the region of the umbilicus in appendicitis. Esophageal pain is frequently confused with that of cardiac origin as they share the same afferent pathways.

A given spinal segment supplies a visceral area with autonomic nerve fibers (afferent and efferent) and also a well-delineated area of the skin (dermatome)

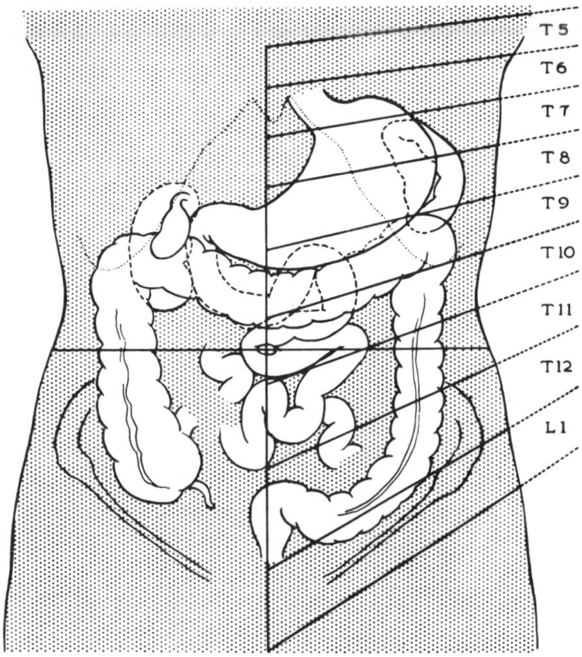

Fig. 13. The segmental distribution of the cerebrospinal nerves from the anterior and lateral parietal surfaces corresponds closely with the dermatomes and represents the same segments of the spinal cord receiving afferent visceral impulses. Smith and Rivers (1953) Peptic ulcer: Pain patterns, diagnosis and medical treatment, Courtesy of Appleton-Century Croft, Inc

with somatic nerves. The two types of structures, linked in this way through the afferent nerves and the central nervous system, may be far apart (e. g., diaphragm, shoulder) or more closely related (e. g., area of abdominal wall and underlying abdominal viscus). Both the splanchnic and cerebrospinal nerve cell bodies are located in the dorsal root ganglia. Here the splanchnic and cerebrospinal cell bodies lie side by side. There proximal fibers also terminate in close proximity within the spinal cord. It is thought that this proximity of the neurons of the two pathways probably accounts for the fact that at times a severe visceral pain seems to "spill over" into somatic segments where it is perceived during the peak of pain. It should be remembered that the spinal segments that supply the dermatomes of the anterior abdominal wall (T-6–L-1) are the same that supply the major portion of the intestinal tract as shown in Fig. 13. The anatomic relationships of the sympathetic and cerebrospinal afferent pathways are shown in Fig. 14.

Although visceral and somatic pain have separate afferent pathways and are appreciated differently by the patient, they frequently occur together.

15.2.4 Shifting Pain

Visceral pain is poorly localized, usually not as severe as somatic pain, and is usually experienced in the midline of the abdomen. The shifting of the pain or a change in the quality of the pain can be of great clinical significance. A classic example is that of the pain of carcinoma of the pancreas. It usually begins as a dull, constant, aching, or gnawing sensation in the upper abdomen but then shifts to the back into the thoracic area. When the visceral pain is very severe, it may spill over at the spinal cord level so the patient now perceives the pain as different and as if it had shifted to a segmental dermatome supplied by the cerebrospinal pathway.

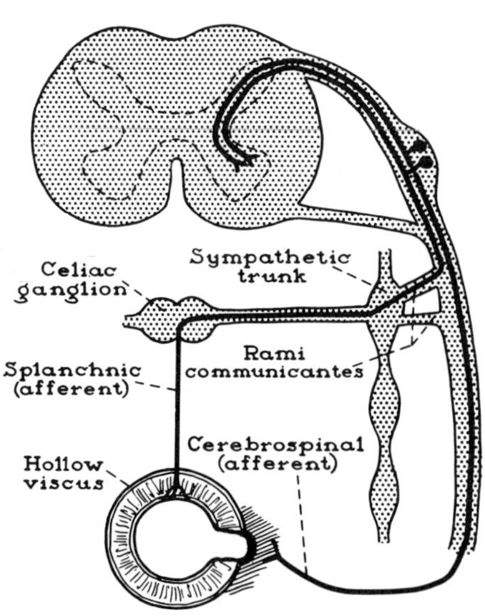

Fig. 14. Afferent splanchnic and cerebrospinal pathways from a hollow viscus and its nearby peritoneum. From Smith and Hanson, An atlas of pain patterns 1961. Courtesy of Charles C Thomas, Publisher, Springfield, Illinois

As the pathologic process causing the visceral pain progresses, it may involve the visceral serosa or the mesentery supplied with somatic nerves, and the location and quality of the pain may shift. Visceral pain may continue, but a new and different pain is now appreciated by the patient.

Sometimes, visceral pain is minimal or is ignored by the patient, who may appreciate the discomfort only when structures innervated by somatic nerves become involved since somatic pain is usually more severe than visceral pain. Thus, the patient and the physician may not suspect that the abdominal pain is of enterocolic origin.

15.3 Abdominal Pain Patterns

Smith and Rivers (1953) almost 30 years ago provided us with an appreciation of specific pain patterns in enterocolic diseases. They pointed out that the clinical correlation of symptoms, anatomic relationships, and surgical findings indicated clearly that the interpretation of the various pain patterns resulting from abdominal lesions could be clarified and properly used at the bedside. From the clinical standpoint, they considered the components of the pain pattern to consist of the location of the primary pain and its shift as well as the quality and behavior of the pain with reference to whether it was acute, chronic, episodic, or unremitting. They also considered important the factors that could precipitate or relieve the abdominal pain. Finally, they considered the severity of the pain and the patient perception, depending on the patient's individual pain threshold.

15.3.1 Location of Pain

Since visceral pain is usually experienced in the midline of the abdomen, the initial site of the pain may give a clue to the site of the pathologic process causing the pain. In general, visceral pain originating in the stomach, duodenum, pancreas, liver, and biliary tree is transmitted to thoracic T-6, T-7, and T-8 and is felt in the midline of the epigastrium. Pain arising from the small bowel below the ligament of Treitz and the proximal colon to the hepatic flexure enters at T-9 and T-10 and is usually felt in the periumbilical area, whereas pain arising in the distal sigmoid colon and rectum enter the cord at T-11, T-12 and L-1 and is usually experienced in the midline of the suprapubic area.

When visceral pain is combined with a somatic element, the location of origin is often easier as the patient usually has tenderness to palpation directly over the diseased organ or tissue.

The position of the patient may influence her interpretation of the exact location of this abdominal distress. For example, when sitting, the patient may indicate that the discomfort is epigastric. However, if she stands or lies flat, she may then indicate the location of the pain by pointing to the hypogastrium.

The shifting of an abdominal pain to a different area may also be of clinical significance. Pain shifting to the right lower quadrant should suggest appendicitis, an ileocecal lesion, Crohn's disease of the terminal ileum, or possibly an inflammed Meckel's diverticulum. Although unusual, pain shifting to the right lower quadrant can be caused by a leaking duodenal ulcer or a lesion in the mesocolon. A shift to the left lower quadrant suggests a lesion in the distal colon or sigmoid, such as diverticulitis. Some unusual causes of left lower quadrant shift include gastric ulcer, pancreatic lesion, or gastrojejunal ulcer (Smith et al. 1961).

15.3.2 Duration of Pain

Consideration should be given to the duration of the patient's pain. When acute, severe, or disabling, the patient will usually seek medical aid early. Thus, the pain may have been present for only a few hours, or a few days at most, when the physician first sees the patient. On the other hand, if the pain is dull and not severe and the patient can tolerate it without too much interference of usual life style or pattern of activities, she might not consult a physician for weeks or even months. Undoubtedly, the patient's tolerance of abdominal pain depends a great deal on her individual pain threshold. Some patients can tolerate little discomfort while others will endure the chronic pain of bowel cancer for months.

Most conditions that cause abdominal pain usually produce pain for a relatively short time. The patient with peptic ulcer pain soon learns that eating or taking an antacid will provide relief. The pain of biliary colic or acute pancreatitis, although frequently severe, lasts only hours or a few days at most.

Abdominal pain, either intermittent or continuous, that lasts 2–3 months is usually considered chronic. In a patient with a chronic steady abdominal pain associated with weight loss, one should always think of the possibility of cancer.

15.3.3 Quality of Pain

Many descriptive terms are used to designate the quality or type of pain the patient is experiencing. Thus, the pain may be described as sharp, cutting, dull, aching, gnawing, severe, constant, pulsatile, intermittent, cramping, griping, spasmodic, burning, colicky, or even explosive. Usually the patient will use a combination of the above or similar terms to describe her pain.

Colicky pain occurring in rhythmic cramps suggests an obstructing lesion in a hollow viscus – usually the gut. Steady pain that varies little from moment to moment indicates a steady stimulus, such as occurs in ulceration of the bowel or an inflammatory process.

Acute severe pain of sudden onset that reaches its full intensity almost immediately suggests an intra-abdominal catastrophe, such as perforation of a viscus or a sudden vascular occlusion.

Lower abdominal cramping, coming on usually after eating and associated with constipation or diarrhea and occurring intermittently for periods of weeks or months for many years duration and not associated with weight loss, suggests the irritable bowel syndrome.

15.4 Enterocolic Disorders Causing Lower Abdominal Pain

It is sometimes difficult to determine if lower abdominal pain is of gynecologic or enterocolic origin. The reason is that the cervix as well as the uterus and its adnexa share the same afferent visceral pathways to the spinal cord as afferent impulses from the lower ileum, colon, sigmoid, and rectum. They all enter at the T-10, T-11, T-12, and L-1 segments of the spinal cord, (Bonica 1953). Thus, the situation is very similar to the problem of chest pain when attempting to differentiate that of cardiac origin from that of esophageal origin (Hightower 1969).

The more common pathologic processes that may cause lower abdominal pain of entercolic origin include a neuromuscular disorder, such as occurs in the irritable bowel syndrome, infectious diarrheas, inflammation, obstruction, tumors, and vascular disorders.

15.4.1 Irritable Bowel Syndrome

The irritable bowel syndrome (IBS) is probably the most common cause of lower abdominal pain seen by the general practitioner as well as the gastroenterologist. Abdominal pain is the predominant symptom in IBS, occurring in 95% of the patients. Associated symptoms include excess gas, diarrhea, and constipation. The pain is usually intermittent and crampy but may be constant. Ritchie has recently stated that the duration of the pain may last only a few minutes in about 30% of patients, a few hours to a few days in 50%, and weeks or longer in the remaining 20% (Ritchie 1979).

The pattern of the pain is rather characteristic. It usually comes on after meals, occurs intermittently for periods of weeks or months for many years duration, and is not associated with any weight loss.

Recent evidence indicates that the colon of patients with IBS is not only more sensitive to distention causing pain but also that the myoelectric activity of the colon in these patients is different from that found in the normal colon.

When a balloon is placed at least 20 cm into the pelvic colon and its volume increased by inflating it by increments, it has been found that normal individuals can tolerate a 60-ml volume without discomfort, whereas approximately 50% of the patients with IBS that were studied experienced pain by the time this volume was reached as shown in Fig. 15 (Ritchie 1977).

When the myoelectric activity of the colon of patients with IBS is recorded, it is found that they have an abnormally high incidence of low-frequency, tone-maintaining electric slow waves (Snape et al. 1977). This increase in the potential reactivity of the bowel persists even when all symptoms of IBS are in remission (Taylor et al. 1978).

The diagnosis of IBS is based upon obtaining a history consistent with the natural history of the disorder, the recognition that symptoms are usually worse during periods of life stress and emotional tension, and the exclusion of other diagnoses that possibly might explain the patients' symptoms (Almy 1973). The clinical pictures usually encountered include the spastic colon with left lower quadrant pain, a persistent painless diarrhea, and alternating diarrhea and con-

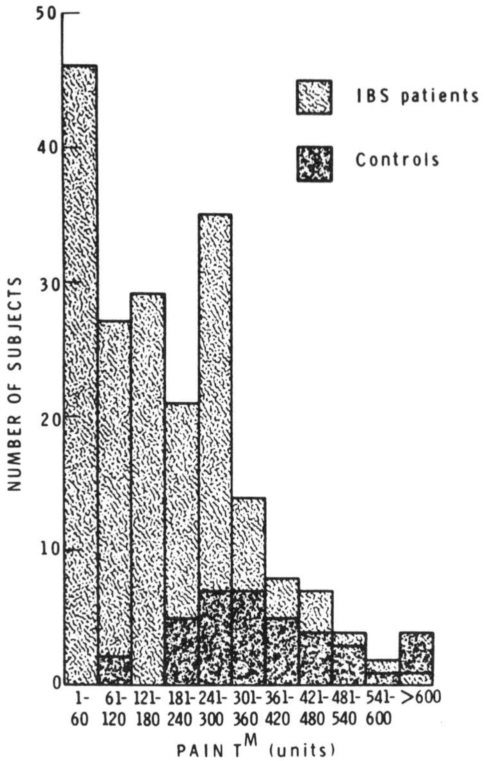

Fig. 15. Histogram showing the number of patients with irritable bowel syndrome and normal controls who experienced pain from balloon distention in the pelvic colon when inflated to different volumes. Ritchie J (1977) The irritable bowel syndrome: manometric and cineradiographic studies. Gastroenterol 6:622–631

stipation. Sigmoidoscopy is usually negative but may show mucosal hyperemia and excess secretion of mucus. The barium enema roentgenogram is usually negative but may show rapid filling, diffuse narrowing, and increased haustra contractions in some patients, while in others there may be a loss of haustration, as is commonly seen in the chronic laxative abuser.

Treatment of IBS, which is usually a lifelong disorder, consists of reassuring the patient that there is no serious gastrointestinal disease present, especially cancer, which is a common fear these patients have, and attempting to teach the patient not only to accept the fact that she has an "irritable" bowel but must learn to live with and cope with the symptoms. Anticholinergic agents will reduce the prolonged postprandial colonic spike and motor response in these patients (Sullivan et al. 1978) The therapeutic efficacy of these agents, however, is still unclear because of the lack of controlled clinical trials. A trial of anticholinergic therapy in a patient with IBS seems justified as some do obtain symptomatic relief. Most authorities also advocate a high-fiber diet in these patients.

15.4.2 Infectious Diarrheas

Infectious diarrheas resulting in acute gastroenteritis are due to a number of enteropathogenic bacteria that produce diarrhea and abdominal cramping because they invade the mucosa, produce an enterotoxin, or both. The intestine reacts to enterotoxins by hypersecretion and hypermotility. This results in the abdominal cramping, which at times can be quite severe.

Shigella invade the intestinal mucosa and some forms, such as *Shigella dysenteriae-1,* also produce an enterotoxin that causes ileal hypersecretion. Characteristic of *Shigella* infection is severe lower abdominal cramps. In addition, the patient will have blood and pus in the stool and considerable tenesmus. Shigellosis usually occurs in epidemic form, particularly in institutionalized subjects. It is usually self-limiting as it rarely lasts longer than 1 week. Usually only supportive treatment is required. In severe cases, if an antibiotic is to be used, ampicillin is the drug of choice.

Enterotoxic *Escherichia coli* is a common cause of traveler's diarrhea. Typically, the diarrhea is of sudden onset, profuse and watery, and accompanied by abdominal colics. The disease is self-limiting, rarely lasting more than 4–5 days, and the patient is afebrile. In adults, no antimicrobial therapy is indicated.

Salmonella gastroenteritis is caused by the endotoxins these bacteria produce. The disease is usually mild and limited to a 1–4 day period. Its main features are lower abdominal cramping or diffuse abdominal colic associated with diarrhea. The disease has a short incubation period and results from the consumption of contaminated food or water. *Salmonella* enteritidis is the most common organism identified. The history is crucial to diagnosis. The patient is usually one of a group who has become ill as a result of ingestion of contaminated food or water. Usually only supportive treatment is required.

Clostridium perfringens is the most widely distributed bacteria that is pathogenic for man. In 1969, in the United States, *C. perfringens* was responsible for more outbreaks of food poisoning than either *Salmonella* or *Staphylococci* (Grady and Keusch 1971). The illness produced by type A *C. perfringens* is self-limited and nonfatal.

Gastroenteritis caused by staphylococci is most often due to the hemolytic *Staphylococcus aureus.* In addition to abdominal colic, the patient usually has nausea and vomiting as well as perfuse watery diarrhea. Gastroenteritis is of short duration and rarely lasts more than 24 h. The cause of the disease is from ingesting food that has been contaminated with staphylococci and has either been inadequately heated or inadequately refrigerated.

Only recently has *Campylobacter fetus* ssp. *jejuni* been recognized as a major enteric pathogen. In a retrospective study, Skirrow (1977) was able to isolate the organism in 7% of 803 patients with diarrhea in 1977. More recently, Blaser et al. (1979) were able to culture the organism in 5% of patients with diarrhea. Abdominal pain is the dominant feature. Tenesmus is uncommon and the diarrhea may not be severe. Associated symptoms include the early onset of fever, headache, and myalgia. The sigmoidoscopic picture resembles that of ulcerative colitis. Both erythromycin and doxycycline have been found effective in treating patients with *C. fetus* infections.

Although human illness caused by *Yersinia enterocolitica* was first described in

New York State in 1933 (Gilbert 1933), infections due to *Y. enterocolitica* are observed and reported much more frequently in western Europe than in the United States. The excellent report by Vantrappen et al. (1977) describes the clinical manifestations of *Y. enterocolitica* infections in man. In a 4-year period, they observed 37 adult patients in their gastrointestinal unit at the University of Leuven in Belgium. The most common symptom was abdominal pain occurring in 84%. The pain was usually described as colicky and was localized in the right iliac fossa in 40% of the patients. The pain was diffuse over the abdomen in 24% and periumbilical in another 8% Diarrhea was the next most common symptom, occurring in 78%, with three to ten watery stools per day and lasting usually 1–2 weeks. Fever was present in 43% of the patients. Anorexia, weight loss, nausea, vomiting, and headache were less common symptoms. Diagnosis was made by isolation of the organism from the stool and by the serum titers of *Yersinia* antibodies. Radiologic signs included abnormalities of the mucosal pattern of the terminal ileum in 67% of the patients. Thus, *Y. enterocolitica* infection must be considered in the differential diagnosis of Crohn's disease of the terminal ileum. Recently, Black et al. (1978), reported an epidemic of *Y. enterocolitica* infection in schoolchildren in the United States due to contaminated chocolate milk served in the school's cafeteria. In these children, the clinical picture closely resembled that of appendicitis, and 16 of the 36 children reported had appendectomies. Vantrappen's group reported that 80% of the positive stool cultures in their laboratories were from children under 10 years of age. When treated with tetracycline or chloramphenicol, symptoms usually disappear in 2–4 weeks.

15.4.3 Appendicitis

Most physicians would probably agree that the abdominal pain of appendicitis is probably the best recognized of the clinical conditions that present with an acute abdomen. The patient usually consults the physician within 12–48 h after onset of symptoms. Over 95% of the patients will have abdominal pain that is most often well-localized in the right lower quadrant (Mittelpunkt and Nora 1966; Sethi et al. 1970). The pain of acute appendicitis is usually first referred to the periumbilical area and later shifts to the right lower quadrant. In approximately 90% of patients, the symptoms of anorexia, nausea, and vomiting will be present.

Renaer and Guzinski (1978) recently pointed out that the physician seeing a young woman with acute lower abdominal pain apparently thinks of "appendicitis" first and may not consider the possibility of the pain being of gynecologic origin. In support of this, they cite the fact that Gilmore et al. (1975) showed that approximately one-quarter of all appendices removed as an emergency procedure were normal and that some 20% of the incorrectly diagnosed conditions were of gynecologic origin. Appendicitis is equally as common in young men as in young women (Green and Watkins 1946). However, Lee has reported that of 18000 appendectomies performed in a series of hospitals of the British National Health Service, there were 7500 more appendectomies in young women between ages 14 and 21 than in young men (Lee 1961).

15.4.4 Diverticulitis

Diverticular disease of the colon is common in the Western world and has been reported to be rare in so-called underdeveloped countries (Painter 1970). In England, for instance, Manousos et al. (1967) carried out a radiologic survey on healthy subjects in the Oxford area and found that diverticula of the colon were present in about 8% of the adult population under the age of 60, whereas in individuals over the age of 70 the incidence was 40%. Necropsy data indicate the presence of diverticula in 50% of patients over 60 years of age, and pathologic evidence of diverticulitis was found in as many as 12% of patients with diverticulosis, although the majority of them had no prior history suggestive of diverticulitis (Hughes 1969).

Diverticulitis is a complication of diverticulosis and results from the perforation of one or more diverticula, causing a pericolitis or a pericolonic abcess. The principal symptoms are lower abdominal pain, usually localized in the left lower quadrant, and fever. Diverticulitis should be strongly suspected in a patient with known diverticulosis who has left lower quadrant pain, fever, leukocytosis, and a tender palpable mass in the left lower quadrant. Sigmoidoscopy without using air insufflation should be done to rule out other conditions; however, a barium enema is contraindicated in the acute phase of diverticulitis. The signs and symptoms of inflammation will usually subside in a few days with treatment, and a barium enema can then be performed safely. The pericolonic abcess often causes ileus or partial or complete colonic obstruction with secondary abdominal distention, anorexia, and nausea.

Treatment consists parenteral administration of appropriate combinations of antibiotics, such as penicillin, ampicillin, and tetracycline, to cover the normal bowel flora. If nausea, vomiting, and abdominal distention are present, nasogastric suction is indicated with appropriate intravenous fluids.

The clinical picture of inflammation involving a Meckel's diverticulum is essentially the same as that of acute appendicitis. Most often, complications of a Meckel's diverticulum occur in young children under the age of 3. The most common symptom is intestinal bleeding due to ulceration of the ileal mucosa by ectopic gastric tissue in the diverticulum.

15.4.5 Inflammatory Bowel Disease

Inflammatory bowel disease (IBD) usually presents in one of three forms: proctosigmoiditis, chronic ulcerative colitis (CUC), or granulomatous disease, of the ileum and/or colon (Crohn's disease).

Proctosigmoiditis is an ulcerative condition involving the mucosa and submucosal structures of the rectum and sigmoid. The proctoscopic picture is identical to that of ulcerative colitis. Patients with ulcerative proctosigmoiditis are characteristically older than patients with ulcerative colitis. Farmer (1979a) has reported that the mean age at the time of diagnosis is 40 years. The principal symptoms are lower abdominal cramping and diarrhea with rectal bleeding associated with tesnesmus and rectal urgency. Farmer (1979b) has found that the prognosis is benign for most patients with ulcerative proctosigmoiditis and in fact has reported that in about 90% of patients, the condition will resolve or remain stable. When proctitis alone exists, the chance of it spreading to the sigmoid colon over a 10-year period is about 30% and to the entire colon 5%–10% (Ritchie and Lennard-Jones 1976). Diagnosis is made by the typical proctoscopic picture and the absence of disease above the sigmoid colon as shown on the barium enema. Treatment of proctosigmoiditis with steroid retention enemas appears to be effective and safe.

Chronic ulcerative colitis (CUC) is also an ulcerative disease of the mucosa and submucosa. The confinement of the pathologic process to these layers of the colonic wall accounts for the patient's inability to accurately or sharply localize her abdominal pain. CUC is more frequent among females than males. It is also predominantly a disease of whites with a higher incidence in Jews. The incidence of cases has been reported to be from 40–80/100000 population.

Ulcerative colitis is a disease that is highly variable. The clinical course may be mild or severe and at times fulminating. Diarrhea is the principal symptom associated with lower abdominal cramping. Rectal bleeding may be minimal or massive. Most patients have an intermittent course with exacerbation lasting a few weeks to a few months, and then remission occurs during which time the patient may be completely asymptomatic. About 10% of patients after an initial attack will have no subsequent symptoms for up to 15 years. Another 10% of patients have continuous symptoms after the onset of their illness with no remissions. In addition to lower abdominal cramping and bloody diarrhea, the patient may also have, depending upon the severity of the disease, fever, anorexia, weight loss, and mild anemia.

The diagnosis of CUC is made by the typical proctoscopic picture and the findings on the colon roentgenograms. Treatment of CUC depends upon the severity of the disease. However, most patients respond satisfactorily to medical therapy when corticosteroids or salicylazosulfapyridine (Azulfidine) are used. Surgical therapy is indicated for certain complications of CUC or when the patient fails to respond to medical therapy.

Granulomatomy disease (Crohn's disease) of the bowel may involve the ileum, especially the terminal portion, the colon, or both organs. Pathologically, Crohn's disease differs from CUC in that it is a transmural disease affecting all layers of the bowel. Intestinal fistulas are much more common in Crohn's disease; perianal abcesses and fistulas occur in up to 70% of patients.

When Crohn's disease is limited to the terminal ileum, it is frequently referred to as regional enteritis. The principal features of the disease are diarrhea, which is accompanied by fever, and right lower quadrant pain. Anorexia, nausea, and vomiting may also be present. There is usually tenderness in the right lower quadrant, and a firm, irregular mass may be palpated. At this stage of the disease, regional enteritis is often mistaken for appendicitis, and the diagnosis is not made until after laparotomy. The disease is chronic, with the patient having periodic exacerbations separated by periods of partial remission. In most patients, however, the process is gradually progressive, and the relative asymptomatic intervals become shorter and shorter.

In granulomatous disease of the colon, there are a number of clinical features that differentiate it from chronic ulcerative colitis. The rectum may be spared in granulomatous disease, whereas in CUC the rectum is universally involved.

Associated small bowel disease occurs in only about 5% of patients with CUC, whereas it is present in approximately 80% of granulomatous colitis. "Skip areas" in CUC are extremely rare, while they occur in about 50% of patients with granulomatous colitis. Perianal disease is three times more common in granulomatous colitis than it is in CUC. On the other hand, carcinoma of the colon is about three times more common in CUC than granulomatous colitis.

Granulomatous disease of the colon occurs most often in the age group from 25–35 years and is slightly more common in females. A patient with granulomatous colitis may first present herself with a complication of the disease, such as a perianal or perirectal abscess and fistula, symptoms of intestinal obstruction, or symptoms of an intra-abdominal fistula or abscess. Fever is a common sign as is gradual weight loss and mild to moderate anemia. Whereas rectal bleeding dominates the course of CUC, it is rare early in the course of granulomatous disease. Approximately one-half of the patients will complain of crampy, colicky lower abdominal pain.

Diagnosis is usually made by barium enema and a small bowel study when the patient has a compatible history. Colonoscopy is also useful in establishing the diagnosis. Medical treatment is similar to that of CUC, and surgery is reserved for dealing with the complications of the disease.

15.4.6 Obstruction

Lower abdominal pain in women can be due to obstruction of the large or small bowel causing either acute, chronic, or chronic pain with acute exacerbations depending upon the degree of obstruction and the rapidity of onset. The pain produced in this situation results from traction on the bowel wall and distention of the bowel lumen. Most obstructions of the bowel are related to adhesions. Adhesions may occur postoperatively, or be due to previous inflammatory reaction in the peritoneal cavity. One large series indicated that postoperative adhesions were responsible for 60% of acute and chronic bowel obstruction. The next most frequent factor was hernia causing 26%, volvulus causing 12%, and mesenteric thrombosis causing 2% (Davis and Sperling 1969). Tumors both benign and malignant do cause bowel obstruction but are relatively infrequent.

The clinical manifestations of intestinal obstruction are abdominal pain, vomiting, and the failure to pass gas or feces. Explosive diarrhea can be present and usually means a partial obstruction. Abdominal distention may vary depending upon the obstruction level and is usually a later symptom. Severe cramping pain is usually diffuse and poorly localized but may be felt in the upper abdomen in patients with high obstruction, at the level of the umbilicus in those with low ileal obstruction, in the lower abdomen in those with colonic obstruction, and in the perineum and lower abdomen in patients with rectosigmoid obstruction. The time period between attacks of pain is 3–5 min with high obstructions and about 10–15 min in patients with low intestinal obstruction. Steady generalized abdominal discomfort will occur when obstruction is not relieved, and distention may become extreme. The severe steady pain with no quiescence accompanied by muscle guarding or rigidity is indicative of strangulation (Hedberg and Welch 1971) and is ominous.

The occurrence and extent of vomiting depends upon the site of obstruction, and with high obstruction vomiting is more frequent. It may not, however, occur for 1 or 2 days in patients with low small bowel obstruction. With high obstruction, the vomitus is copious and may effectively decompress the bowel. In lower intestinal obstruction, it is frequently malodorous and feculent. Vomiting is usually not present with colonic obstruction but will occur in the case of an incompetent ileocecal valve.

Auscultation is of great value in the diagnosis of a simple mechanical obstruction in that bowel sounds are quiet except during attacks of colic when sounds become loud, high-pitched, and metallic and occur in rushes. In patients with chronic recurring partial bowel obstruction, these signs and symptoms may occur spontaneously or in the course of a disease causes some edema of the bowel walls, such as an acute viral illness. The attacks may be very mild, requir-

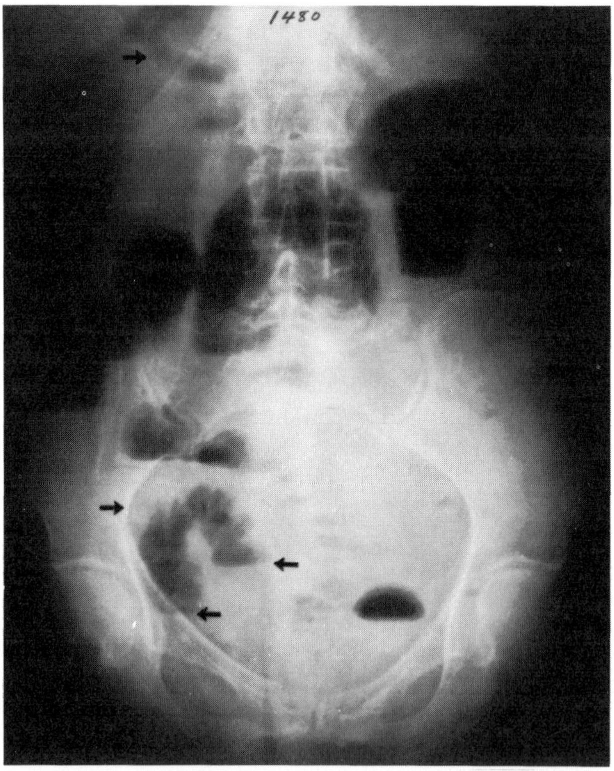

Fig. 16. An example of differential air-fluid levels *(arrows)* as observed in acute mechanical obstruction of the small bowel. Note that the air-fluids levels occur at different levels when the roentgenogram is obtained in the upright position. In this case, the obstruction was caused by a large gallstone *(arrow)* at the ileocecal valve. Air is also seen in the biliary tree at the top of the film

ing only that the patient refrain from ingestion of food for a few hours and are spontaneously relieved. Such attacks, however, usually are recurrent and eventually will lead the patient to seek medical attention for relief of the pain and obstruction.

Laboratory findings in patients with intestinal obstruction depend upon the severity of the obstruction. Patients who have a low-grade partial small bowel obstruction with lower abdominal pain and no distention or vomiting usually have no positive laboratory findings. In patients who, however, are suffering from an acute attack, the hematocrit level usually rises in proportion to the amount of fluid sequestered in the bowel or lost with vomiting. The urine-specific gravity may be elevated and is important in determining the severity of the dehydration that has occurred. In early stages of obstruction, there is little change in the concentration of sodium, potassium, or chloride in the plasma; however, in untreated long-standing intestinal obstruction, dehydration with loss of electrolytes may be severe. Patients who have had recurrent episodes of lower abdominal pain, thought to be related to intermittent obstruction, should be watched very closely when an acute exacerbation of their pain occurs so that strangulation of the bowel with subsequent perforation will not be allowed to develop.

Diagnostic procedures are of importance and should include roentgenograms of the abdomen. Plain films should be obtained in the supine, left lateral, and upright positions. Posteroanterior and lateral views of the chest should also be obtained. Differential air fluid levels in the small bowel are diagnostic of mechanical obstruction as shown in Fig. 16. There are several other conditions in which air fluid levels may be observed in the bowel, including adynamic ileus, extreme aerophagia, gastroenteritis, severe constipation, and sprue (Ellis 1971). These conditions, however, will not be associated with a differential air fluid levels. Additional radiologic studies, such as barium enema, intravenous pyelogram (IVP), and administration of contrast material orally or through a nasogastric tube, may be indicated. With colonic obstruction, a barium enema may provide information on the type and location of the obstruction; however, there are dangers in the barium enema studies, particularly in inflammatory lesions, such as diverticulitis, which may lead to possible perforation. Forcing barium past a partially obstructing lesion may also cause the formation of inspissated barium followed by a complete obstruction. A dilute barium solution given orally or through a nasogastric tube if necessary will help to diagnose the type of intestinal obstruction or locate the precise areas of simple mechanical obstruction in patients who have small bowel obstruction. If the contrast material can be seen throughout the entire intestinal tract, the diagnosis of complete obstruction is ruled out. One, however, may see chronically distended small bowel with edema in the wall, matting loops of small bowel in the pelvis, and areas with poor peristalsis under fluoroscopy, which would lead one to make the diagnosis of a chronic partial small bowel obstruction. An IVP may locate ureteral calculi, which often produce paralytic or adynamic ileus and is useful in evaluation of patients with lower abdominal pain of undertermined etiology.

Treatment

After the diagnosis of an acute intestinal obstruction has been made, if the patient has been adequately hydrated with replacement of electrolyte deficiencies and treated with nasogastric suction and antibiotics, a decision must necessarily be made whether or not surgery is indicated. If strangulation obstruction is suspected and the patient is febrile with an elevated white count, then early surgery is definitely indicated. In patients who have the syndrome of lower abdominal pain, constant or recurrent, with acute exacerbations in whom a diagnosis of intermittent partial small bowel obstruction is made, the indications for surgery are somewhat less distinct. It is our practice to ask these patients when they have an acute exacerbation of their abdominal pain to come to the hospital even in the middle of the night to the emergency room for evaluation. If indeed the syndrome is full-blown enough that a diagnosis of partial small bowel obstruction is made and this has been a recurrent problem with the patient over several months to years, we feel that exploratory laparotomy with lysis of adhesions is indicated. If at the time of surgery, one adhesive band is found, then no additional surgery is indicated. If, however, there are multiple adhesions involving the large and small bowel, then internal plication with a Baker tube is the treatment of choice (Nadrowski 1974). The reason for the plication is that we do know that these adhesions will reform and when they do it is hoped that the internal plication will allow them to form in a manner that will not cause kinking of the bowel with subsequent recurrent pain and obstruction.

15.4.7 Tumors

Tumors of the gastrointestinal tract can and do cause chronic lower abdominal pain in women and by necessity should be considered in the diagnostic evaluation and differential diagnosis of chronic lower abdominal pain in women. Tumors of the small bowel are relatively uncommon. Benign tumors, such as leiomyomas and hamartomatous polyps, and malignant tumors, such as adenocarcinomas, lymphomas and carcinoids, are usually diagnosed at the time of exploratory laparotomy for either chronic or acute small bowel obstruction. Because they are relatively high in the gastrointestinal tract, the pain that they cause is usually upper to midabdomen and does not fit within the scope of this discussion. Tumors, however, of the colon, especially the sigmoid and the rectum, do frequently cause lower abdominal pain. Tumors, such as adenomatous polyps, villous tumors, adenocarcinomas, carcinoids, lymphomas, melandomas, and leiomyosarcomas, all can be the etiologic agent in lower abdominal pain in women. Most tumors, benign or malignant, do not cause acute or even chronic pelvic pain until they reach a far advanced stage, causing either obstruction of the bowel or the invasion of pelvic organs with resultant torsion or hemorrhage (Localio and Eng 1975).

The most frequent and first symptom of neoplasia of the rectum and sigmoid is a change in bowel habit. Constipation and diarrhea or a combination of these is reported in approximately 75% of patients. The next most frequent symptom is abdominal pain, which occurs in approximately 65% of patients. Weight loss and rectal bleeding with abdominal distension are also prominent symptoms in advanced disease, and at this point in time a lower abdominal mass can usually be palpated (McSherry et al. 1969).

On physical examination, a large number of rectal tumors can be palpated by rectal and vaginal examinations. With large tumors, invasion of the pelvic structures may be present, which can be demonstrated by fixation of the pelvic organs to the palpable abdominal mass. Proctoscopic examination should be performed on these patients and is positive in a large percentage. Biopsy of the tumor should be accomplished when it can easily be visualized. Barium enema examinations are also useful in these patients, both to show the size and the extent of the tumor and to rule out other intracolonic neoplasms.

Treatment

Patients with large rectal and sigmoid malignancies should have these tumors removed. Often it is necessary to remove the pelvic organs at the same time because of contiguous spread. Our philosophy of this problem includes the attempted removal of all neoplasms in this area. We feel that patients are best palliated by removal of the tumor mass as opposed to biopsy and proximal diverting colostomy followed by postoperative radiation.

15.4.8 Pelvic Abscess

Acute peritoneal infections usually follow a pattern determined by anatomic disposition of the organs and tissues. The so-called abdominal watershed is formed by the mesenteric attachment of the small bowel from the left upper to the right lower quadrant. Extravasation to the right of this line follows the gutter to the right lower quadrant. Those to the left follow the usual course to the pelvis (Hau et al. 1979). Pelvic abscesses are probably the most common type of localization following generalized or local peritonitis or open bowel operations of any sort. The apparent collection accumulates in the most dependent portion of the peritoneal cul-de-sac where it may be detected at a very early stage by pelvic and/or rectal examination. Larger abscesses may present anteriorly in the suprapubic region or may extend upward and laterally in either direction to the iliac or even to the paracolic gutter. Of all the intraperitoneal abscesses, the pelvic abscess is perhaps the only one that can usually be regarded as a beneficial development.

Pelvic abscesses may be suspected in patients with lower abdominal pain, anorexia, fever, and the findings of a tender mass on pelvic or rectal examination (Franklin et al. 1973). As the pelvic abscess becomes more chronic, the patient may not manifest fever, and the pain pattern may become more of a constant low-grade pelvic pain with acute exacerbation reminiscent of a chronic small bowel obstruction. Diagnostically, roentgenograms of the abdomen will not demonstrate the presence of an abscess unless it causes significant distortion or displacement of adjacent structures or if extraluminal gas can be identified. Unfortunately, the significance of extraluminal gas is difficult to evaluate in abscesses, especially in the early postoperative period. Beta mode ultrasound scanning in the determination of intra-abdominal abscesses has been reported to be quite accurate (Wolson 1977). The ultrasound does not depend upon indirect signs but rather clearly outlines the fluid collections, demonstrating both the size and the location of the abscess. It is even more beneficial in patients with chronic pelvic abscess or patients who have had recurrence of pelvic abscesses in that it will demonstrate these graphically, documenting the recurrence at the original site as opposed to a new location, or will demonstrate multiple abscesses should they be present. Computerized axial tomography also is an excellent way to demonstrate the presence of a pelvic abscess, but our experience has been very limited to date.

It must be recognized that pelvic abscesses from whatever origin will secondarily involve the female genital tract and may progress to salpingitis, pyosalpinx, and usually involve the ovary (McNamara and Mead 1976). The clinical determination of the precise character of the inflammatory pelvic mass, the pelvic abscess, is not possible unless all cases are subjected to early surgical intervention.

Although local irritation of the rectum may cause diarrhea, the systemic signs and symptoms seem less marked than with other abscesses in higher parts of the abdomen, and there is also perhaps less tendency to intestinal obstruction since the small bowel loops tend to float over the purulent accumulation. It is often difficult to distinguish a pelvic phlegmon or cellulitis from an actual abscess formation since both may present as a tender pelvic mass with systemic signs of toxemia. These cellulitises may subside gradually without treatment although antibiotics would doubtless be recommended in every case. Similarly, true collections of pus may resolve spontaneously either by absorption or by rupture into the rectum or posterior vaginal fornix (Hedberg and Welch 1971).

Abdominal pain, rectal tenderness, bladder irritation, or small bowel involvement constitutes a relative indication for surgical intervention. In a patient who is moderately or markedly toxic, the indication for drainage after a period of observation is even more pressing. Although there is still some controversy about the timing and the need for surgery to drain pelvic abscesses, the following indications seem reasonable: (1) an abscess amenable to drainage by posterior colpotomy or other extraperitoneal route, (2) abscess refractory to conservative management, that is, the absence of defervescence or increasing in size of the mass in the pelvis, (3) cases in which the diagnosis of acute unruptured pelvic abscess is questionable, and (4) presence or suspicion of a ruptured pelvic abscess. It should be emphasized strongly that even though surgical drainage of a pelvic abscess may be indicated on the basis of systemic effects, this mass should nevertheless not be approached through the rectum or the vagina unless there is very definite evidence of fluctuation. If the mass has neither softened in the rectum or enlarged to the extent that it may be palpated suprapubicly, it may be better to wait for further developments while maintaining the patient on antibiotic coverage. It is interesting that many of these masses that at first seem certain to drain into the bowel may either disappear spontaneously initially or later present suprapubicly or in an iliac position. Any attempt to hurry the process by rectal or vaginal incision runs the risk of unnecessary disruption or contamination of a slowly resolving phlegmon or, even worse, a useless injury to a loop of small intestine. When fluctuation does become apparent, the surgeon may then safely proceed with rectal or vaginal drainage under general anesthesia. Conservative therapy is appropriate for patients who do not demonstrate recognized abdominal rigidity and rebound tenderness at the time of admission or during the course of the initial medical therapy and who demonstrate a response by general defervescence without signs of increase of the pelvic mass and optimally accompanied by a decrease in the size of the pelvic mass during the initial 48–72 h of therapy.

It has been found by adopting this conservative approach to the treatment of pelvic abscesses that the pregnancy rate in these patients is extremely low. In addition, further surgery is required in a high percentage of these patients at a later date as dictated by symptoms of recurrent pelvic abscess, chronic pain, or small bowel obstruction (Franklin et al. 1973). On the basis of these findings, some authors advocate early radical surgical treatment, including total abdominal hysterectomy and bilateral salpingo-oophorectomy with drainage in essentially all patients with true pelvic abscesses whether they arise from within the female genitalia or from an extragenital route. We feel, however, that this approach is unduly aggressive and that initially a conservative management should be tried. When we are dealing with a chronic pelvic abscess that has not evolved into a fluctuating collection in the pouch of Douglas or persisted after a posterior colpotomy, unilateral or symmetric pelvic tenderness is usually found and an indurated cul-de-sac without fluctuation into the rectum. Because the superior margin of the abscess usually involves the small bowel, there may be signs of intermittent small bowel obstruction. It is our policy when such an abscess can positively be identified and the patient is significantly symptomatic that an exploratory laporotomy be done with lysis of adhesions of the small bowel and removal of the pelvic visceral organs with drainage through the vagina. The overall result of this form of therapy is excellent.

15.4.9 Hernias

In the differential diagnosis of lower abdominal pain in women, hernia is often excluded because of the relatively low incidence of hernias in females as opposed to males. The other obvious problem in making the diagnosis in the female is that the female usually is placed on the examining table either in the supine or lithotomy position, and the hernia that she has will be in a reduced state and therefore undiagnosable.

There are three hernias of the groin that occur in the female, the most frequent being that of an indirect inguinal hernia followed by a direct inguinal hernia and also the femoral hernia. The indirect inguinal hernia is congenital in origin and develops as a failure of the spontaneous closure of the vaginal process, which allows for intra-abdominal contents to protrude through the internal inguinal ring into the inguinal canal. The direct inguinal hernia, which frequently occurs in adults past the age of 40, develops as a weakening of the transverse fascia in Hesselbach's triangle area and is felt to be acquired. The femoral hernia, which is a hernia more common in women than in men, emerges through the femoral canal under Poupart's ligament and presents itself at the saphenous opening. Femoral hernias are quite rare before the age of puberty and are a disease of adult life. In spite of this, many authorities regard the sac as being a congenital prolongation of peritoneum through the femoral canal (Koontz 1963). Unquestionably, exertion, straining, and coughing play a contributory role, as a great many elderly people develop femoral hernias.

Symptoms of inguinal hernias can be quite varied depending upon the size of the hernia and whether or not incarceration or strangulation is present. Often the complaint stated to the physician is the finding of a mass either in the groin or just below the inguinal ligament; this may be completely asymptomatic or found by the physician as part of a routine physical examination. Often, however, the strain of lifting will cause a painful feeling in the inguinal region, which may be referred into the lower abdomen; once the hernia is fully developed, there may be a sense of a weighty discomfort in the groin and the lower abdomen on that side. If the hernia becomes strangulated, the usual signs of intestinal obstruction appear and are associated with a tender and irreducible mass in the area. The patient should be examined in a standing position. If a mass is present either in the inguinal area or below Poupart's ligament, an effort should be made to reduce it and the size of the ring determined. If it is not reducible with the patient standing, she should be examined in the recumbent position to determine whether the hernia is reducible and if so to determine the size of the ring. Often, hernias cannot be reduced in the office but will reduce themselves during the night, and a history of this can be obtained. It is not infrequent that a femoral hernia will present as an intestinal obstruction due to strangulation. Often, the presence of the femoral hernia is unknown both to the patient and to the patient's doctor. Even after the strangulation occurs, diagnosis of an intestinal obstruction is made, the cause of which is not known. The surgeon called in such cases should always look for a femoral hernia, especially in women. In fat women, the hernia is often not visible because of the fat but is readily palpable as a hard mass in strangulated cases.

Sometimes, the gynecologist will encounter a patient who has a typical history compatible with a hernia and on examination no hernia can be found. This does not definitely rule out the presence of a hernia, and it may require subsequent examinations to prove this. It is better to examine the patient after she has been on her feet for prolonged periods of time as opposed to the early morning when the hernia has been reduced all night. After the patient has been standing at her job all day, the hernia frequently is much more readily diagnosable than it is in the morning. If a hernia can be demonstrated in the groin, then proper surgical repair will effect a cure in the vast majority of patients.

Primary perineal hernias can also be the cause of lower abdominal and perineal pain in women. Perineal hernias are the rarest of all hernias and occur five times more frequently in women than in men. Most cases occur between the ages of 40 and 60 years. The pathologic process involves the floor of the pelvis, which is formed by the levator ani and the coccygeus muscles and their fascia. Perineal hernias emerge through openings or defects in this floor. There are two main types, the anterior and the posterior. The anterior type emerges anterior to the transverse perineum and is said to occur more frequently in males. The anterior type will generally present in the labia majora in the female. The posterior type emerges posterior. In the anterior type, the bladder is often contained in the wall of the sac. Symptoms related to the anterior hernia are a painful enlargement in the area of the labia. The pain may be referred into the pelvis. The posterior type emerges posterior to the transverse perineum and comes through the pelvic floor, either through the levator ani muscle itself or between the levator ani and the coccygeus muscles. It is most frequently observed in the female. It generally emerges halfway between the rectum and the tuberosity of the ischium. Intestine and omentum are commonly reported contents of the sac in the posterior perineal hernias, and the symptoms are related to localized pain in the area and sometimes a great deal of discomfort when the patient tries to sit down. The pain may be referred into the low abdomen. On examination, the soft reducible mass is characteristic. The direction along which the mass is reduced determines the nature of the hernia. If there is bladder in the sac, as is often the case in the anterior variety, the percussion notes over the hernia are dull. This is also true if omentum is in the sac. When the sac contains bowel, as is frequently the case in the posterior type, the percussion note may be tympanitic. In rare cases of strangulation, the mass may be swollen, tender, painful, and completely irreducible, at which point signs and symptoms of intestinal obstruction with abdominal pain and distention will develop. The presence of a reducible mass in either of these areas makes the diagnosis. With bimanual, rectal, or vaginal examination, disclosure of a mass that can be pushed up into the cul-desac of Douglas will confirm the diagnosis. Differential diagnosis of this condition includes lipomas and fibromas, all of which form masses that are not reducible.

The only rational treatment is operation. Supports of any kind are worthless. The operation should be done through an abdominal route because the defect can be closed more easily and the contents of the sac may be dealt with in a more reasonable fashion. The abdominal route is mandatory in the case of a strangulation.

An obturator hernia is a rare type of hernia that protrudes through the obturator foramen. This hernia is six times more frequent in women than in men, probably due to the broader female pelvis, larger obturator foramen, and the stresses of pregnancy and childbirth. The peak age, for instance, is 50 years of age. They are more common in thin people with a history of recent weight loss. Apparently, the loss of fat in the obturator canal is a predisposing cause. Other predisposing causes are coughing or straining and other causes of increased intra-abdominal pressure.

The hernia sac protrudes through the obturator foramen along the course of the obturator vessels and nerves. It is usually just lateral to them. The sac lies mesad to the femoral canal and usually presents itself under the pectineus muscle. The most frequently found contents of the sac are small intestine. Large intestine, however, may also be found. Omentum is rarely found. Ovaries, tube, and appendix and part of the uterus have been reported to be in the sac in unusual cases. The symptoms may not be present, and a mass may be palpated in the medial aspect of the thigh, but the most common symptoms of a nonstrangulated hernia consist of pain in the sensory distribution down the inside of the thigh due to pressure on the obturator nerve by the hernial mass. Gastrointestinal symptoms, such as abdominal pain, constipation, nausea, vomiting, and colic, may also be present. Symptoms of intestinal obstruction may offer the first clinical signs and are a result of incarceration of the hernia. It sometimes may be difficult to differentiate this from a femoral hernia; however, it is much more medial and beneath the pectineus muscle and in thinner people should be readily differentiated from a femoral hernia.

As with previous hernias discussed here, surgical approach is required and should be done from the abdomen. The contents of the sac are reduced and dealt with according to their state of viability, and the sac is drawn out by grasping the fundus with a clamp and pulling it inside into the abdominal cavity. It is ligated at the neck and either excised or folded on itself and sutured into place to plug the opening in the obturator canal. The obturator canal is difficult to close because of the rigidity of the environs. A piece of Marlex mesh may be needed to completely obliterate the hernial space.

15.4.10 Intestinal Ischemia (Abdominal Angina)

Inadequate intestinal blood flow may result in functional derangements or impair the structural integrity of the bowel. Included under the heading of chronic intestinal ischemia are those conditions in which there is insufficient blood flow to satisfy the demands of increased motility, secretion, and absorption that develops after meals. These disorders manifest themselves by either ischemic visceral pain and/or abnormalities in gastrointestinal absorption or motility. Patients with chronic intestinal ischemia are actually experiencing recurrent acute attacks of insufficient blood flow during periods of maximal intestinal work loads. Therefore, the pain is similar to that arising in the myocardium during angina pectoris or in calf muscles with intermittent claudication.

Chronic intestinal ischemia has been reported with aneurysms of the aorta, celiac axis, and superior mesenteric artery, with congenital and traumatic arterial venous fistulas involving the superior mesenteric artery and hepatic arteries, with coarctation of the aorta, and with congenital anomalies of the splanchnic vessels (Boley et al. 1978). Such cases are rare, however, and arteriosclerotic involvement of the mesenteric vessels is almost always the cause of this form of intestinal ischemia. This atherosclerotic process commonly involves the splanchnic arteries in individuals over 45 years of age. Although this abnormality has commonly been found in patients at autopsy, the frequency of the syndrome of chronic intestinal ischemia has been seen in relatively few patients.

15.4.10.1 Clinical Features

The one consistent clinical feature of chronic mesenteric ischemia is abdominal discomfort or pain. Most commonly this occurs 10–15 min after eating, gradually increases in severity, reaches a plateau, and then slowly abates in 1–3 h. The pain is most often cramping in nature. It is located most frequently in the upper abdomen but can be pelvic in nature and radiate into the back. Initially, the pain occurs only after large meals, but characteristically there is progressive increase in both the frequency and the severity of attacks with time. The pain pattern is so intimately related to the ingestion of food that the patient will reduce the size of meals, become reluctant to eat, and even develop frank cibophobia. The result of this is significant, and often massive weight loss, bloating, flatulence, and derangements in the motility with constipation and/or diarrhea occur. Intermittent episodes of vomiting occur much less commonly. Steatorrhea with "stool floating in the water" is observed by approximately one-half of these patients.

Physical findings are both limited and nonspecific. The patient, however, will appear chronically ill and show signs of marked weight loss. This should be a tip-off to the gynecologist evaluating such a patient with lower abdominal pain. The abdomen is usually soft and nontender even during episodes of pain, and there may be some distension observed. A systolic bruit is heard over the upper abdomen in approximately one-half of these patients (Boley et al. 1978). Many patients will have a history of physical manifestations of associated cardiac, cerebral, or peripheral vascular insufficiency.

15.4.10.2 Diagnosis

There is no specific viable diagnostic test for abdominal angina at this time. The diagnosis must be based on the clinical syndrome and the angiographic demonstrations of the occlusive process of the splanchnic vessels with the exclusion of other gastrointestinal and gynecologic disorders. Conventional radiographic examinations of the gastrointestinal tract and pelvic examination are usually unremarkable. The roentgenograms, however, may reveal evidence of decreased motility in the form of puddling of barium in the jejunum. Studies for malabsorption may show increased fecal fat, decreased urinary excretion of D-xylose, and less often increased fecal nitrogen. Although these tests identify absorption defects, none are specific for malabsorption due to ischemia. Abnormalities have been detected in small bowel biopsies, but again there is nothing specific for ischemic disease. Occult blood in the stools is present usually at some stage in the disease process.

Angiographic evaluation including flush aortography in the frontal and lateral views and subsequent injections of the superior mesenteric and celiac axis and if possible inferior mesenteric artery are indicated (Boley et al. 1978). The degree of occlusive involvement of the three major arteries can best be assessed on the lateral projections. A collateral circulation and flow are best seen in the frontal views. The presence of prominent collateral vessels indicates a significant stenosis of a major vessel and also quantitates a chronic process. Angiographic demonstration of stenosis or occlusion of one or two or all of the major vessels does not by itself establish a diagnosis of arterial insufficiency.

With no available methods for measuring intestinal blood flow, precise criteria to define the need for operative arterial reconstructions are lacking. There is agreement that the patient with atypical pain of abdominal angina and unexplained weight loss, with diagnostic evaluation having excluded other gastrointestinal and gynecologic disease, and with arteriograms that show occlusive involvement of at least two of the three major arteries should have benefit of operation (Boley et al. 1978).

At present, the preferred procedure for atherosclerotic occlusive or stenotic disease of the celiac axis and superior mesenteric artery is a bypass from the aorta to the superior mesenteric artery. The procedure is designed to provide rapid exposure and to facilitate the performance of the anastomosis.

References

Almy TP (1973) Irritable colon. In: Gastrointestinal disease. Pathophysiology, diagnosis, management. Sleisenger MH, Fordtran JS (eds). Saunders, Philadelphia, pp 1278–1288

Bentley FH, Smithwick EH (1940) Visceral pain produced by balloon distention of the jejunum. Lancet II:389

Black RE, Jackson RJ, Tsai T, Medvesky M, Shayegani M, Feeley JC, MacLeod KIE, Wakelee AM (1978) Epidemic Yersinia enterocolitica infection due to contaminated chocolate milk. N Engl J Med 298:76–79

Blaser MJ, Berkowitz ID, LaForce FM, Cravens J, Reller LB, Wang WL (1979) Campylobacter enteritis: clinical and epidemiologic features. Ann Intern Med 91:179–185

Boley SJ, Brandt LJ, Veith FJ (1978) Ischemic disorder of the intestines. Curr Probl Surg 15:1–85

Bonica JJ (1953) The management of pain. Lea & Febiger, Philadelphia

Davis SE, Sperling L (1969) Obstruction of the small intestine. Arch Surg 99:424–426

Ellis H (1971) The cause and prevention of postoperative intraperitoneal adhesions. Surg Gynecol Obstet 133:497–511

Farmer RG (1979a) Long term prognosis of patients with ulcerative proctosigmoiditis (ulcerative colitis confined to the rectum and sigmoid colon). J Clin Gastroenterol 1:47–50

Farmer RG (1979b) Prognosis and management of proctosigmoidit. Pract Gastroenterol 3:44–52

Franklin EW III, Henron JE Jr, Thompson JD (1973) Management of the pelvic abscess. Clin Obstet Gynecol 16:66–79

Gilbert R (1953) Interesting cases and unusual specimens. Annual Report of the Division of Laboratory Research. Albany, New York, New York State Department of Health, p 57

Gilmore OJA, Browett JP, Griffin PH, Ross IK, Brodribb AJM, Cooke TJC, Higgs MJ, Williamson FCN (1975) Appendicitis and mimicking conditions. Lancet II:421–424

Grady GF, Keusch GT (1971) Pathogenesis of bacterial diarrheas. N Engl J Med 285:831

Green HW, Watkins V (1946) Appendicitis in Cleveland; final report. Surg Gynecol Obstet 83:613–624

Hau T, Ahrenholz DH, Simmons RL (1979) Secondary bacterial peritonitis: the biologic basis of treatment. Curr Probl Surg 16:1–65

Hedberg SE, Welch CE (1971) Suppurative peritonitis with major abscesses. In: Hardy JD (ed) Critical surgical illness. Saunders, Philadelphia, pp 436–476

Hightower NC (1969) Applied physiology of the esophagus. In: Paulson M (ed) Gastroenterologic medicine. Lee & Febiger, Philadelphia, pp 19–39

Hightower NC, Janowitz HD (1978) Innervation and visceral sensations of the gastrointestinal tract. In: Brobeck JR (ed) Best and Taylor's physiological basis of medical practice. Williams & Wilkins, Baltimore, 2.13–2.19

Hughes LE (1969) Postmortem survey of diverticular disease of the colon. I. Diverticulosis and diverticulitis. II. The muscular abnormality in the sigmoid colon. Gut 10:334–336

Hurst AF (1911) The sensibility of the alimentary canal. Frowde, London

Koontz AR (1963) Hernia. Appleton-Century-Crofts, New York

Kuntz A (1953) The autonomic nervous system, 4th edn. Lea & Febiger, Philadelphia

Lee JA (1961) Appendicitis in young women. Lancet II:815–817

Localio SA, Eng K (1975) Malignant tumors of the rectum. Curr Probl Surg 1–48

Manousos ON, Truelove SC, Lumsden K (1967) Prevalence of colonic diverticulosis in the general population of Oxford area. Br Med J 3:762

McNamara MT, Mead PB (1976) Diagnosis and management of pelvic abscess. J Reprod Med 17:299–304
McSherry CK, Cornell GN, Glen F (1969) Carcinoma of the colon and rectum. Ann Surg 169:502–509
Mittelpunkt A, Nora PF (1966) Current features in the treatment of acute appendicitis: an analysis of 1000 consecutive cases. Surgery 60:971
Nadrowski LF (1974) Pathophysiology and current treatment of intestinal obstruction. Rev Surg 31:381–407
Painter NS (1970) Diverticular disease of the colon-a disease of Western civilization. DM 3:57
Renaer M, Guzinski GM (1978) Pain in gynecologic practice. Pain 5:305–331
Ritchie J (1977) The irritable bowel syndrome: manometric and cineradiographic studies. Clin Gastroenterol 6:622–631
Ritchie J (1979) Pain in irritable bowel syndrome. Pract Gastroenterol 3:16–23
Ritchie JK, Lennard-Jones JE (1976) Crohn's disease of the distal large bowel. Scand J Gastroenterol 11:433–436
Sethi SM, Matsuda T, Pemberton LB, Strohl EL (1970) An analysis of 500 consecutive cases of acute appendicitis in a metropolital charity hospital. Ill Med J 138:147
Skirrow MB (1977) Campylobacter enteritis; a (new) disease. Br Med J II:9–11
Smith LA, Rivers AB (1953) Peptic ulcer: Pain patterns, diagnosis, and medical treatment. New York, Appleton-Century-Crofts, p 576
Smith LA, Christensen NA, Hanson NO, Ralston DE, Achor RW, Berge KG, Morrow GW Jr, Bulbulian AH (1961) An atlas of pain patterns. Sites and behavior of pain in certain common diseases of the upper abdomen. Thomas, Springfield, p 54
Snape WJ Jr, Carlson GM, Matarazzo SA, Cohen S (1977) Evidence that abnormal myoelectrical activity produces colonic motor dysfunction in the irritable bowel syndrome. Gastroenterology 72:383–387
Sullivan MA, Cohen S, Snape WJ Jr (1978) Colonic myoelectrical activity in irritable bowel syndrome. N Engl J Med 298:878–883
Taylor I, Darby C, Hammond P, Basu P (1978) Is there a myoelectrical abnormality in the irritable colon syndrome? Gut 19:391–395
Vantrappen G, Ponette E, Geboes K, Bertrand PH (1977) Yersinia enteritis and enterocolitis: gastroenterological aspects. Gastroenterology 72:220–227
Wolson AH (1977) Ultrasound diagnosis of pelvic and wound abscess after an appendectomy. Surg Gynecol Obstet 144:376–380

16 Low Back Pain in Women (E. Morscher)

16.1 Introduction

About 80% of all people suffer from back pain at some time in their lives. Women are no more frequently affected than men. In their case, however, problems in differential diagnosis are more numerous because of particular anatomic and physiologic factors. Patients with back pain account for 6.5% of those in a gynecologic practice (Hackenbruch et al. 1979). The cause of low back pain may be gynecologic, vascular, neurologic, psychogenic, or spondylogenic. Spondylogenic pain, which will be our main concern here, originates in

the axial skeleton and its structures. It is characteristic of this pain that it is usually related to physical activity. Its origin can be in the bones, the intervertebral disks and small intervertebral joints, the soft tissues, or the back muscles. The latter have a particularly important role since the ultimate cause of low back pain in most cases is decompensation, static or dynamic, of the spinal and pelvic structures, which play active and passive parts in support and movement.
There are two reasons why low back pain is so common: (1) the lumbosacral junction is the point where the mobile part of the vertebral column joins the rigid pelvic part and (2) this is the part of the spine that carries the greatest mechanical load. Man's upright posture is fundamentally responsible for both these important circumstances.

16.2 Definition of Low Back Pain

Low back pain is merely a symptom. The doctor's task is to discover its cause so that rational and, if possible, specific treatment may be given. The first essential is to distinguish chronic, though usually intermittent, lumbago from acute low back pain (also called acute lumbago). Pain radiating from the small of the back to the leg is usually called sciatica by the patients themselves. Sciatica must be distinguished from so-called root irritation, a less well-defined radiating pain unaccompanied by objective neurologic signs (pseudoradicular pain).

16.3 Medicosocial Importance of Low Back Pain

As already mentioned, 80% of people suffer from low back pain at some time in their lives. Unander-Scharin (1950) found the highest incidence of low back pain in women aged 35–45 years. According to Severin (1944), 70% of patients with low back pain seek medical advice before they reach the age of 45 years. Of women in Sweden between 15 and 71 years of age questioned by Hirsch et al. (1969), about one-half reported some kind of back pain. These figures confirm the medicosocially important fact that women are particularly prone to low back pain during the years when special demands devolve upon them as mothers and housewives. In most of the developed countries, low back pain causes a loss of time from work of 5% (Nachemson 1978).

16.4 Origin of Low Back Pain

One of the biggest unsolved problems of lumbago is to know where the pain originates. There is, of course, an obvious explanation in some pathologic conditions, such as inflammation, neoplasms, and Baastrup's disease (interspinal osteoarthrosis, „kissing spine"), but even with spondylolisthesis, it can be difficult to say where the pain arises. In a large percentage of cases, the displacement is asymptomatic throughout life or for several decades at least.
The following anatomic structures in the spine may be considered as possible sources of pain:

1) *Muscles* are probably the most frequent sources of pain. They become painful as a result of decompensation or strain and excessive fatigability after exertion. In almost all cases of so-called vertebral insufficiency (however this is caused), they are responsible for the pain.
2) In the early 1930s, Ghormley (1933) focussed attention on the *small intervertebral joints* as sources of pain and spoke of the "facet syndrome." The capsules of these joints are innervated by the posterior roots of the spinal nerves. Badgley (1941) also considered changes in these joints to be important in relation to lumbago and sciatica. More recently, these ideas have been taken up again by Mooney and Robertson (1976), Shealy (1976), and Niethard and Gaertner (1979).
3) After 1934, when Mixter and Barr recognized disk herniation as the main cause of sciatic pain, the *intervertebral disk* became the focus of interest, but here the circumstances causing pain are still far from clear. American orthopedic surgeons in particular saw instability of the motion segment as the main cause of pain in patients with disk degeneration (Mensor et al. 1959; Morgan and King 1957; Lettin 1967). This is now the usual reason for deciding that fusion of a painful and degenerating "motion segment" is indicated. The "motion segment concept" came from Schmorl and Junghanns (1951). It means the functional unit formed by the articular interconnections of two vertebrae, whereby the intervertebral disk and the two facet joints are particularly important. Instability, however, does not explain why patients with disk pain prefer moving to sitting or lying still.
4) That back pain might be caused or explained by *intraosseous* hypertension has been claimed by Arnoldi and his colleagues (1972). Intraosseous venous stasis has often been demonstrated in arthroses at other sites, especially the hip and knee (Arlet and Ficat 1968; Morscher and Friedrich 1971). That an increase or change in pressure in the marrow space can cause severe pain was made clear to us during intraosseous phlebographies when, at first, no anesthetic was given. Moreover, as is well-known, arthrotic pain rapidly subsides after an osteotomy, probably simply because of decrease in pressure in the marrow space. Arnoldi et al. (1972) succeeded in measuring raised intraosseous pressures in the spinous process marrow spaces of patients with lumbago.

16.5 Investigation of Low Back Pain

The investigation of a patient suffering from low back pain embraces (1) history, (2) physical examination, (3) roentgenography, and (4) special laboratory investigations.

16.5.1 History

Although there is no specific pain that is pathognomonic of the etiology of a patient's lumbago, a carefully taken history usually enables a provisional diagnosis to be made. The following questions must be answered as precisely as possible.

16.5.1.1 Localization of Symptoms

In localizing the pain, the term "small of the back" is not adequate. Important differential diagnostic conclusions can often be drawn from an exact description and localization of the pain. The sacrum is usually indicated as the site of pain of gynecologic origin, while patients with spondylogenic pain point more to the lumbosacral junction, the area of the posterior iliac spines, the paravertebral sacrospinalis muscles, or the sacroiliac joints (Fig. 17).

When pain radiating into the legs is complained of, root pain and pseudoradicular pain must be distinguished, the former being confirmed by objective neurologic signs.

Pain in the neighborhood of the sacroiliac joints is associated not only with disorders of these joints themselves but quite frequently also with instability of the pubic symphysis occurring in pregnancy and childbirth (Pechel 1965). Back pain is very often localized not at its site of origin, in other words the site of the offending lesion, but more caudally.

16.5.1.2 Timing and Nature of First Appearance of Low Back Pain

Low back pain that originally occurs after an accident, after physical exertion, or in the morning on rising, or is obviously associated with fatigue, clearly suggests an "orthopedic" genesis. However, spondylogenic pain can also occur for the first time during pregnancy or the puerperium. Nongynecologic low back pain can even abate and intensify in unison with the menstrual cycle. Krupp and Levy (1963) investigated 67 women treated for disk herniation and found that 80% had experienced their first attack when they were of childbearing age, and 16

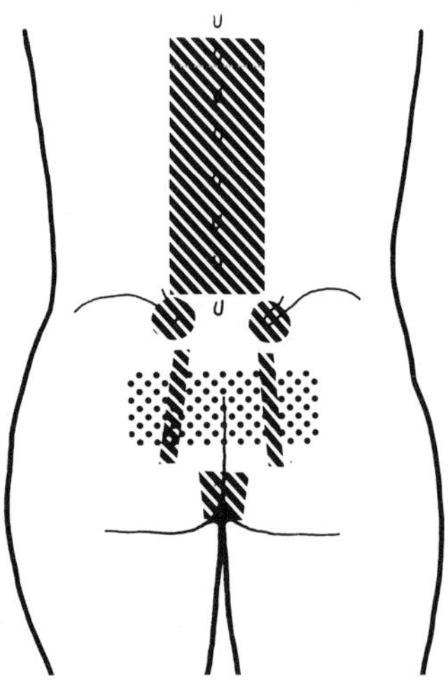

Fig. 17. Localization of low back pain in women

▧ Spondylogenic pain

⁘ Pain of gynecologic origin

(about one-quarter) had first had it during pregnancy, delivery, or the puerperium. One-half of the women had suffered a recurrence of disk herniation during a later pregnancy.
Acute lumbago that comes on during some perfectly ordinary everyday activity, such as getting up from a chair or lifting a heavy object, suggests so-called intervertebral joint blocking.

16.5.1.3 Relation of Intensity of Pain to Time of Day

Spondylogenic pain in a large proportion of cases is a consequence of static and dynamic malfunction of the spine. Therefore, it is often characterized as pain clearly associated with fatigue. This, of course, also applies to the pain occurring with uterine prolapse (Gau 1967), which begins when the patient is fatigued and increases as the day goes on.
Pain that begins during rest and eases during movement is very suggestive of an intervertebral disk disorder. Pain from spondylarthrosis sometimes has the same characteristic.
Deeply situated low back pain that comes on in the night and decreases with movement is suggestive of ankylosing spondylitis, but this condition is more prevalent in males.

16.5.1.4 Relation of Low Back Pain to Posture

The load on the intervertebral disks is greatly influenced by back posture. Nachemson measured directly the pressures in the lumbar intervertebral disks in different body postures. As shown in Fig. 18, the load on the lumbar intervertebral disks is least in the supine recumbent position and greatest in the sitting

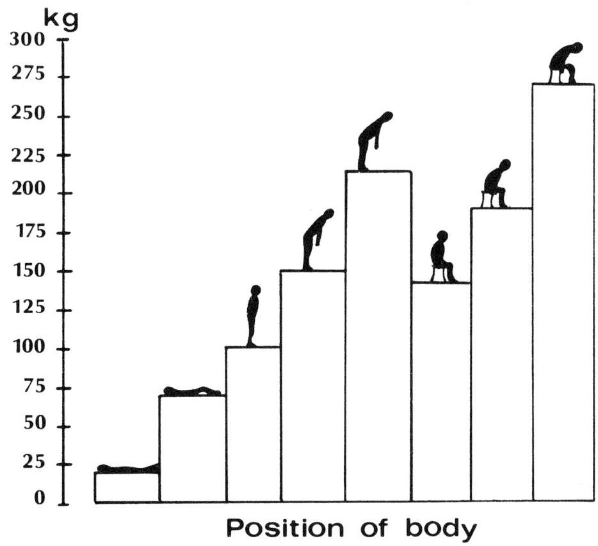

Fig. 18. Relative load on third lumbar disk. In a subject of 70 kg the load in upright standing position is approximately 40 kg (400N). According to Nachemson (1960)

position with the upper part of the body bent forward. Pain commencing during prolonged standing or sitting, especially with the upper part of the body bent forward (sewing, secretarial work, etc.), is therefore suggestive of a disk lesion. Indirectly, it is usually the result of static mechanical insufficiency (muscle fatigue).

16.5.1.5 Previous History and Results of Treatment

Acute lumbago disappears within 3 weeks in 70% of cases, and within 2 months in 90% (Nachemson 1978).

16.5.2 Physical Examination

A systematic routine is just as necessary in conducting the physical examination as it is in taking the history, mainly to ensure completeness but also to save time. The basic essentials of every examination are:

1) *Inspection* of the undressed patient. Particular attention is directed to body build, muscular development, and the configuration of the spine, i. e., the patient's posture.
2) *Examination of function,* with measurement of movements in all directions (flexion and extension, lateral flexion, and rotation in each part of the spine).
3) *Palpation,* mainly of the musculature and the spinous processes. As to the musculature, tone, pronounced tenderness on pressure, and the presence of "myogeloses" are important. The spinous processes are examined for pain on pressure, percussion, or jolting. Pain on jolting is typical of instability of a motion segment or of part of a vertebra, e. g., in cases of spondylolisthesis. Subluxation of the vertebra in the latter condition usually produces a palpable step in the row of spinous processes. Of particular importance – especially in women – is the clinical examination of the sacroiliac joints. Tenderness may be found on pressure over these joints and over the pubic symphysis. In addition, pain can be provoked by movement of these joints, e. g., by lateral compression of the pelvis, forced abduction of the hips (in the absence of hip joint disease, of course), or hyperextension of the hips (Gaenslen's sign).

16.5.3 Roentgenologic Investigation

Although the roentgenogram has a central role in the elucidation of low back pain, a dangerous and often repeated mistake is that of unreservedly accepting the roentgenologic diagnosis as the cause of the patient's symptoms. Roentgenograms sometimes reveal little or nothing abnormal during the initial and most painful stage of a spinal disorder. At a later stage, there is often less pain even though irreversible changes are present and roentgenograms reveal severe destruction.

The most important task when interpreting roentgenographic findings is to correlate them with the clinical symptoms. In general, the correlation is very poor. For example, Reinhard and Heinemann (1964) inspected 3245 roentgenograms from women with low back pain and found that only 7.5% were entirely free from abnormalities (244). Multiple changes were found in 66.5% (2159) and a single abnormality in 26% (842). These and other studies show clearly how wrong it would be to draw direct conclusions about a patient's symptoms from roentgenograms alone.

So-called functional roentgenologic investigation is of special value where the spine is concerned because it provides information about the "soft tissue factor," which is usually far more important in pain causation than the roentgenographically visible skeleton. The following are the principal methods of investigation employed in functional investigation:

1) Evaluating and comparing roentgenograms of the spine taken when the patient is:
   - Lying, standing, and sitting
   - In maximum forward flexion and in maximum extension
   - In maximum lateral flexion to the left and right
2) Study of spinal movements with an automatic cassette changer (Sollmann)
3) Functional tomography (Seidel and Bertram 1974)

As already mentioned, an important role in the causation of low back pain is attributed to instability of a motion segment. Most authors consider that mobility in the sagittal plane is greatest in the L-5/S-1 segment. In contrast, lateral mobility at that site is practically nil. Rotational movements are very difficult to measure roentgenologically. Mobility of the lumbosacral segment may be almost abolished in patients with low back pain, but lack of mobility is also seen in 15% of people with no symptoms, the proportion rising to 43% in subjects with lumbago (Mensor et al. 1959). Instability is most often found in the L-4/L-5 motion segment. It is recognized by the reciprocal anteroposterior displacement of the two vertebrae. Only a positive finding is significant as muscle spasm can prevent displacement even though a segment is unstable.

16.5.3.1 Myelography

Myelography is of most value in the investigation of disk herniation. According to Hirsch and Nachemson (1963), the correlation between myelographic and operative findings is 90%, but myelography should be used more for preoperative determination of the level of a disk lesion than for diagnosis alone.

16.5.3.2 Diskography, i. e., injection of contrast medium directly into the disk, was introduced by Lindblom in 1948. It is now rarely used in the investigation of lumbar risk herniation, though it is still of some value in the diagnosis of cervical disk disorders. One reason for the rather limited diagnostic potential of diskography is apparent from the fact that Holt (1968) found positive diskographic appearances in 37% of asymptomatic subjects.

16.5.4 Special Investigations

A routine investigation in all cases of back pain is measurement of the erythrocyte sedimentation rate. Böhni (1964) used this criterion to divide patients with back pain into two major groups:
1) Those *with* a raised erythrocyte sedimentation rate
2) Those *without* a raised erythrocyte sedimentation rate
The first group includes rheumatic patients and those with back pain of inflammatory or neoplastic origin (metastases). An extremely important investigation, above all in the diagnosis of spinal tumors and inflammations, is *scintigraphy.*

16.6 Etiology of Low Back Pain

It cannot be too strongly emphasized that low back pain is a symptom and not an illness in itself and that quite often the cause is elsewhere than in the spine. The very numerous causes of low back pain have been classified by Macnab (1977) as follows: viscerogenic, vascular, neurogenic, psychogenic, and spondylogenic. Only the last group is considered here. Included in it is the very common "functional back pain." This diagnosis – and incidentally that of psychogenic back pain – should be made only if an organic cause can be excluded. Most cases of functional low back pain are due to muscle weakness or inadequacy, e. g., because of obesity or after parturition. Whenever obesity seems to be a causal factor of "functional back pain," weight reduction is in order. When the back pain is due to weakness of the abdominal muscles after parturition, muscle strengthening exercises under the control of a physiotherapist are indicated.

16.6.1 Congenital Anomalies

The significance of congenital anomalies in the etiology of low back pain is disputed (Nachemson 1971). Examples are spina bifida, sacralization and lumbarization, elongated transverse processes, block vertebrae, and asymmetry of joints (e. g., unilateral facet joint agenesis). The anomalies most likely to cause chronically recurring low back pain are asymmetric transitional vertebrae (hemisacralization, hemilumbarization) (Fig. 19). Another consideration is that where congenital malformations have immobilized one or more motion segments, the neighboring segments will be overloaded and will undergo premature degenerative changes. This also applies to operative fixation of vertebrae (spinal fusion).

16.6.2 Growth Disorders

16.6.2.1 Scoliosis

Scoliosis of major degree is clinically important mainly as a cause of disfigurement and of interference with cardiorespiratory function. As a cause of low back pain it ranks low in order of importance. Obliquity of the pelvis resulting from

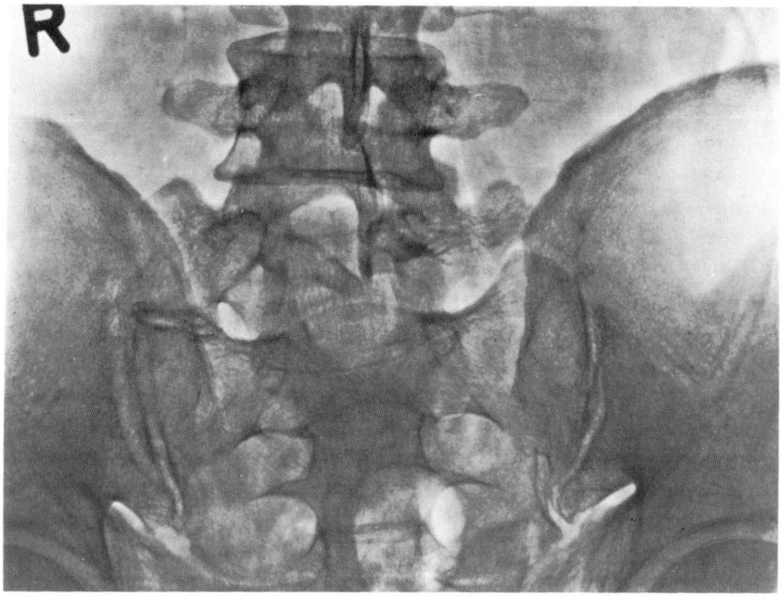

Fig. 19. Asymetric transitional vertebra of the lumbosacral area

inequality of leg lengths is understandably a cause of lumbago. In such cases, the first objective is to equalize the leg lengths.

Leg length can be measured either clinically or roentgenologically. The latter method is almost confined to scientific studies but is sometimes used before operative correction of leg length. Clinical measurement of leg length may be direct or indirect. In the direct method, the distance between the anterior iliac spine and the tip of the external malleolus is measured, while in the indirect method boards of known thickness are placed beneath the shorter leg until the pelvis is horizontal. These two methods of measurement are not alternatives; they are complementary. The tape-measure method determines true length, divided into upper and lower leg lengths if necessary, while functional differences in leg length can be assessed by the indirect method, e. g., when flexion contracture at the hip or knee (or both) is causing functional leg shortening (Morscher and Taillard 1965; Morscher and Figner 1972).

In all cases of lateral curvature of the spine, it is necessary to distinguish between postural scoliosis (which is correctable, as in the instance of pelvic obliquity from leg length inequality) and true structural scoliosis, which is characterized by fixation of the vertebrae in the scoliotic segment, longitudinal torsion of the spine (crowding of the ribs on one side), and roentgenographically detectable anatomic changes in the vertebrae.

Lumbago is much more often associated with lumbar scoliosis than with thoracic scoliosis. Nevertheless, scoliosis is usually overrated as a cause of lumbago. The deformity is distressing, but pain is hardly ever experienced before 20 years of age, and its incidence in adults is not significantly greater than in the general population (Nachemson 1971).

16.6.2.2 Scheuermann's Disease

Another cause of chronic lumbago is Scheuermann's disease and its sequelae. This name is given to a growth disorder of the vertebral column that leads to kyphosis and rigidity in the affected segment. The roentgenographic signs are intervertebral disk narrowing, Schmorl's nodes, and wedging of vertebrae. According to Gschwend (1965), 80% of patients who have been treated for Scheuermann's disease in their youth complain of back pain later in life, the proportion being especially high among those with the lumbar form of the disease.

Scheuermann's disease, like scoliosis, has long been overrated as a cause of symptoms. Ross (1963) found Schmorl's nodes in the roentgenograms of 39% of 5000 healthy police recruits. Rompe (1965) examined spinal roentgenograms from 1000 unselected patients treated in the Heidelberg Orthopedic Hospital and found juvenile growth disorders in the end plates of 69%. It is therefore clear that a single finding, such as a Schmorl's node, is of relatively little significance. Such studies also show how hazy and indistinct the boundaries are between physiologic and pathologic states. Diagnosis and prognosis must always be based on clinical examination with assessment of spinal configuration and spinal mobility in different directions so that ankylosed and still mobile segments are identified as well as on the roentgenographic appearances.

16.6.2.3 Spondylolysis, Spondylolisthesis

Evidence of spondylolysis is found in 5%–7% of our population and of spondylolisthesis in 2%–4%. Although displacement of a vertebra is undoubtedly a significant cause of symptoms, it is also recognized that a large proportion of people with a spondylolisthesis may remain free from pain all their lives.

Following Newman (1963) we distinguish congenital, isthmic (spondylolytic), traumatic, degenerative, and pathologic forms of spondylolisthesis.

Congenital spondylolisthesis is usually due to elongation of the pars interarticularis, although it remains intact. Some cases progress to complete forward dislocation of the body of the fifth lumbar vertebra in front of the sacrum (spondyloptosis).

In isthmic spondylolisthesis, the vertebral arch is interrupted in its interarticular part (spondylolysis). Degenerative spondylolisthesis is caused by degeneration of the intervertebral disk, usually at the L-4/L-5 level. In the great majority of cases, it is possible to alleviate or abolish symptoms and disablement by conservative measures (remedial exercises, corset treatment). Indications for operation (fusion, Fig. 20) are:

1) Pain that cannot be relieved by properly performed conservative measures.
2) Neurologic symptoms or signs. According to De Palma and Rothmann (1969), sciatica may be the only symptom of spondylolisthesis in 12% of cases.
3) An increase in the displacement, which seldom occurs after growth is complete.

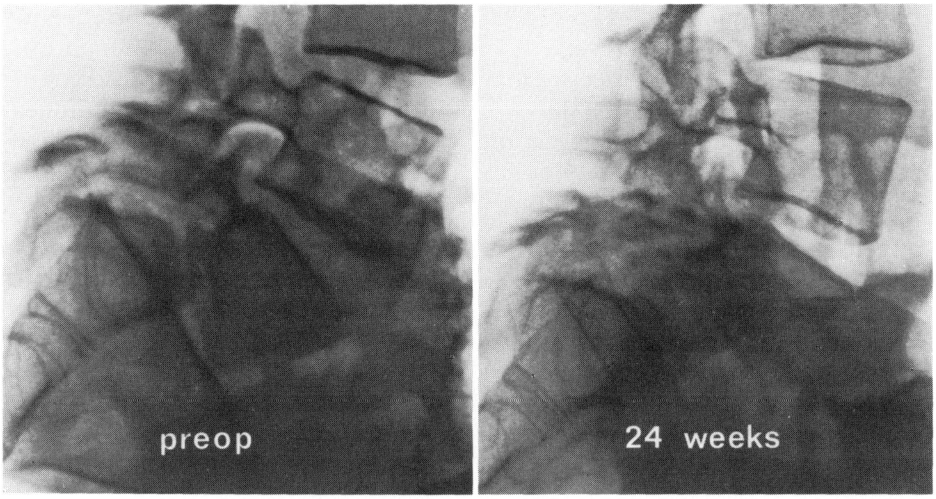

Fig. 20. Anterior fusion of L-5/S-1 intervertebral disk in spondylolisthesis. Note reduction of displacement of vertebra L-5 and enlargement of the intervertebral space by the graft.

4) A relative indication for operation, according to Taillard (1957), is pronounced trapezoidal deformation of the body of the fifth lumbar vertebra, convexity of the upper surface of the first sacral vertebra, and abnormal mobility, i. e., instability, of the affected motion segment. In doubtful cases, considerable occupational demands on the spine should count as an indication *for* rather than against operation.

Spondyloptosis, especially if associated with scoliosis of the spine, may be corrected instrumentally and stabilized by spinal fusion (Harrington and Tullos 1971; Vidal et al. 1973; Morscher 1975).

16.6.3 Traumatic Lesions of the Vertebral Column

Spinal injuries are a common cause of chronic lumbago. Frequently, however, it is not the spinal injury itself that causes pain, but preexisting pathologic changes that become painful when aggravated by trauma. Direct consequences of spinal trauma are instability and changes in spinal mechanics, the latter resulting mainly from compression fractures and fracture dislocations. Here, too, the prognosis is particularly unfavorable if the potential for compensation is limited (Scheuermann's disease, spondylolisthesis). Circumstances can thus arise in which correction of the deformity is indicated. In our experience, corrective osteotomy after recent or old compression fractures is most often indicated in younger patients with severe deformity, poor adaptation potential, and heavy occupational demands on the back (Morscher 1970, 1972).

Injuries that appear unimportant on roentgenographic evaluation, such as avulsion of one or more transverse processes, can cause lasting trouble.

It must be remembered that compression fractures of the spine are frequently overlooked. This applies very much indeed to elderly women with osteoporosis. Back pain after commonplace trauma (lifting a heavy weight), and also constipation and bowel distension by gas (which is caused by a retroperitoneal hematoma), should always suggest the possibility of a spinal compression fracture.

16.6.4 Inflammation

Despite its relative rarity as a cause of back pain, inflammation should invariably be thought of. Spinal infections are always painful. Even so, they often go undetected, at least initially, because some time elapses before any roentgenographic changes appear. In agreement with Macnab (1977), we distinguish the following clinicopathologic syndromes:

1) *Pyogenic vertebral osteomyelitis.* The most common pathogens are staphylococci, *Pseudomonas,* and gram-negative bacilli.
2) *Tuberculous vertebral osteomyelitis.* The thoracolumbar junction is the most usual site. The interval between the onset of symptoms and the establishment of the diagnosis is often remarkably long, not uncommonly extending to several months.
3) *Miscellaneous infections of the spine.* These are caused by a wide range of organisms, such as Brucella, fungi, and parasites, including syphilis.
4) *Intervertebral disk space infection.* The most common cause is surgical ablation of a ruptured intervertebral disk. The sequence of events is characteristic. Infection after a diskectomy must be considered, especially when severe pain recurs after a period of relief lasting a week or several weeks.
5) *Intervertebral disk inflammation.* This is encountered only in children.

16.6.5 Tumors

Neoplasms are a relatively rare cause of back pain, but the pain is usually particularly severe and implacable. The most common primary tumor in the spine is myeloma, exceeded among malignant neoplasms only by metastases. As a source of spinal metastases, by far the most common primary tumor is carcinoma of the breast. The treatment of spinal tumors naturally depends on their nature. Operation is occasionally indicated because of threatened instability and spinal cord compression. Timely active intervention (total excision of a spinal metastasis and operative stabilization) will usually succeed in mobilizing an otherwise bedfast patient and warding off paraplegia.

16.6.6 Osteoporosis

Whether osteoporosis really causes pain is a perennial topic for discussion, and the present view is that it is probably not a direct cause. Kokowski (1965) investigated 416 patients over 45 years of age and could not correlate the roentgenograms to the pain pattern with respect to age incidence of osteoporosis, localization, or degree. The combination of marked osteoporosis and low back pain always calls for a valid clinical explanation. For example, a patient who at first sight seems to have banal osteoporosis with compression fractures may in fact be suffering from myelomatosis.

16.6.7 Postdiskectomy Syndrome

The term "postdiskectomy syndrome" denotes low back pain that continues after a herniated disk has been removed. Residual symptoms after herniated disk operations were noted by Kuhlendahl and Hensell (1953) in 60% of their cases. Bösch (1969) reported that 10–20 years after operation 77% of 151 patients complained of low back pain. Campbell and Newman (1971) collated statistics from 11 studies embracing a total of 3053 laminectomies and found that 1458 patients (47.8%) were left with chronic lumbago. This persuaded many orthopedic surgeons, especially in the United States, to carry out spinal fusion immediately after removing the disk. This practice has now largely been abandoned, partly because spinal fusion does not guarantee lasting freedom from pain and partly because the additional operation is not always necessary. A large-scale inquiry by the American Orthopedic Association showed that in 10% of cases spinal fusion was performed at some time after operation for disk herniation. Pain persisting after disk surgery can have various causes. These include instability of the motion segment after disk ablation, arthrosis of the small intervertrebral joints because of incongruity resulting from collapse and fusion of the disk space, and adhesions (dural or radicular). In the opinion of Brodsky (1976), the main causes of recurrence of root pain, other than another herniated disk, are thickening of the vertebral arch as a consequence of the subperiosteal stripping or of an excess of scar tissue. Furthermore, after the disk has been ablated and the disk space has narrowed, root compression by the superior articular process of the body of the subjacent vertebra is a possibility (Benini 1976).

16.6.8 Degenerative Changes in the Spine

Degenerative changes easily take first place among organic causes of low back pain. Intervertebral disk degeneration probably accounts for about 50% of cases of low back pain.

Among the degenerative conditions to be distinguished are chondrosis, osteochondrosis, spondylosis, and spondylarthrosis.

The features of chondrosis and osteochondrosis, in other words, degeneration of the intervertebral disk, are loss of mucopolysaccharides and dehydration; both these changes cause loss of tensile strength and elasticity in the annulus fibrosus. Roentgenograms simply show disk space narrowing with chondrosis, but in the case of osteochondrosis they also show sclerosis and osteophyte formation in the end plate areas. Spondylosis shows osteophyte formation on the end plates. Osteophytes must be carefully distinguished from "traction spurs" (Macnab

1977), which develop horizontally about 2 mm away from the edge of the end plate and are an expression of instability of the corresponding intervertebral disk. Spondylarthrosis means degeneration of the small intervertebral joints.
A degenerating intervertebral disk may cause pain, but need not necessarily do so. It may cause instability of the motion segment, but again not always. Many American orthopedic surgeons are among those who consider that instability of a motion segment is a frequent cause of low back pain. For example, Mensor (1959) thought it was the cause in 13% of 527 cases of lumbago, and Morgan and King (1957) thougth it was to blame in as many as 28% of patients. Likewise, because of the analogous clinical findings in patients with structural defects and patients with degenerative changes, Lettin (1967) regarded mechanical instability as a cause of low back pain in both groups.
Pain from a prolapsed disk radiating into the legs is usually preceded by intermittent attacks of lumbago over a long period. One of the main indications for disk surgery is an increasing or suddenly appearing neurologic deficit, especially if it affects the bladder and bowel (Bianco 1968). The indication for operation is determined by the neurologic signs, not by the back pain. Insofar as sciatica is concerned, laminectomy for disk herniation is likely to be successful in 90%–95% of cases. As already mentioned, however, chronic lumbago is still to be expected in 40%–50% and a recurrence of sciatica in 5%. "Chronic spinal arachnoiditis" is probably a common cause of pain recurrence after operation.

16.6.9 Spinal Stenosis

Narrowing of the spinal canal as a possible cause of chronic back pain, especially in older patients, has proved of increasing interest in recent years. Verbiest drew attention to this clinical entity in 1948 and reported on 97 cases in 1975.

16.6.10 Pathologic Changes in the Sacroiliac Joints

In the differential diagnosis of low back pain in women, it is especially important to consider the pelvis, and in particular the sacroiliac joints. During the last months of pregnancy, relaxation of the ligaments, induced by hormones, prepares for parturition. During this period, the sacroiliac joints are highly vulnerable and strain is easily caused, even by trivial stresses. The typical signs of "sacroiliac sprains" have been defined by Macnab (1977) as pain on resisted abduction of the hip, pain on bearing weight on the affected side, pain on pressure over the pubic symphysis, and a positive Trendelenburg's sign. A "very tight webbing belt" worn between the iliac crests and the trochanters is usually effective.
True instability of the sacroiliac joints is caused by severe trauma with disruption of the pelvic girdle. Reactive changes at the pubic symphysis can often be seen in roentgenograms, and dislocation can be demonstrated when the patient stands on either leg alone.
Inflammatory conditions to be considered are ankylosing spondylitis and then psoriasis and Reiter's disease. The slightest suspicion of ankylosing spondylitis

should always lead to inquiry for a history of swollen or painful joints, urethritis, iritis, pain in the heels, and of course any relevant family history.
Among infections, tuberculosis used to be preeminent, but pyogenic infections of the sacroiliac joints now appear to be more frequent. The least suspicion of inflammation of the sacroiliac joints is an indication for scintigraphy, but it must be remembered that an elevated uptake in their neighborhood is physiologic. Nevertheless, a "hot spot" may be a clue leading to correct diagnosis.

16.6.11 Coccygodynia

The differential diagnosis of coccygeal pain is peculiarly difficult. Women are more prone to coccygodynia than men. The 115 patients reported on by Buchmann (1966) included 94 women aged between 11 and 60 years. Trauma was blamed in 52% of cases. It is well-known that psychological factors are of exceptional importance in coccygeal pain, far more so than in lumbago. Whenever no definite cause for the pain can be found, it is therefore best to withhold treatment as far as possible, especially massage, other kinds of physical treatment, and operation in particular. Just using a cushion when sitting is sometimes helpful. It is an established fact that such complaints, which are frequently functional in origin, eventually disappear even without any treatment. Coccygectomy certainly requires great circumspection, as all too often it does more harm than good.

16.6.12 Pubic Symphysis Pain

Affections of the pubic symphysis are a not uncommon cause of pelvic pain in everyday gynecologic practice. Probably foremost among these is instability of the pubic symphysis associated with childbirth. The cardinal signs are painful restriction of abduction of both legs and limitation of rotation at both hip joints, pain on pressure over the pubic symphysis, separation of the pubic bones in some cases, and pain in the neighborhood of the sacroiliac joints on moving the hip joints. Apart from instability or separation of the pubic symphysis after childbirth, the following conditions are encountered from time to time and should be thought of: tuberculosis of the pubic bones and pubic symphysis, pubic osteomyelitis, pubic osteitis, posttraumatic pubic osteonecrosis, ankylosing spondylitis affecting the pubic bones, and posttraumatic changes in the pubic symphysis (Spranger 1972).

16.7 General Rules of Treatment and Conduct for Patients with Back Complaints

Apart from specific therapeutic procedures appropriate to the diagnosis, the management of back pain calls for certain general measures that are applicable in all cases. These measures help to prevent fresh attacks of pain, especially in cases of chronic recurrent lumbago. They comprise physiotherapy, attendance at a "low back school," and social intervention in matters such as employment counseling, alteration of working procedures, change of occupation.

Remedial gymnastics occupy a central place in the management of low back pain, but active exercises are much more valuable than passive movements. It is imperative that the patient should carry out the exercises regularly. The question of whether – and if so, when – the patient should wear a belt or corset is not always easy to answer. One absolute indication is the aftertreatment of spinal fusion; another is serious instability of the spine, e. g., after laminectomy and in cases of vertebral fracture due to osteoporosis. The condition known as "vertebral insufficiency" is merely a relative indication. In such cases, it is much better for the patient to build up his or her own "muscle corset" by regular and intensive exercises. The "low back school" has two aims: (1) to give the patient some understanding of the cause and nature of the complaint and (2) to restore his or her confidence. It is essential that the patients grasp the purpose of the measures prescribed by the doctor so that they can collaborate actively in their own recovery. Such training is the surest way of preventing neurotic fixation and perpetuation of back pain. There are many people who complain of back pain not because they are psychopathic, but whose continuous suffering has made them nervous and irritable.

Every patient with back pain must strictly obey certain rules of conduct. Patients must know what they ought to do and what they should avoid. In brief summary, here are the rules and precautions with which every patient should be familiar:

- Assume a flat position in bed at night
- Engage in an appropriate sport: swimming (if lordosis is painful, as in spondylolisthesis, swimming on the back is recommended)
- Know the right way of getting out of bed; when tying the shoelaces, and in other such operations, the spine must be kept flat, i. e., extended
- Use proper seats and chairs
- When sitting (office chairs, car seats), keep the spine extended, e. g., by a lumbar support if necessary
- Emply the correct methods of lifting: keep the spine extended, thus ensuring uniform loading of the intervertebral disks and maintenance of reserves of elasticity
- Avoid lifting heavy loads
- Carry loads close to the body's center of gravity
- Lift weights with the legs and not the back
- Distribute loads symmetrically (use two shopping bags instead of one)
- Use mechanical aids for lifting
- Avoid sudden jerks when lifting
- Avoid twisting movements of the loaded spine
- Avoid long periods of work in one position (e. g., washing up, ironing, etc.); prolonged bending forward is particularly harmful
- Avoid vertical shocks or jarring of the spine (vehicles with poor shock absorbers, high heels).

References

Arlet JP, Ficat P (1968) Diagnostic de l'ostéonécrose fémorocapitale primitive au stade I (Stade préradiologique). Rev Chir Orthop 54:637–648

Arnoldi CC, Lemperg RK, Linderholm H (1971) Immediate effect of osteotomy on the intramedullary pressure of the femoral head and neck in patients with degenerative osteoarthritis. Acta Orthop Scand 42:357–365

Arnoldi CC (1972) Intervertebral pressures in patients with lumbar pain, Acta Orthop Scand 43:109–117

Arnoldi CC, Linderholm H, Müssbichler H (1972) Venous engorgement and intraosseous hypertension in osteoarthritis of the hip. J Bone Joint Surg [Br] 54:409–421

Badgley EE (1941) The articular facet in relation to low back pain and sciatic radiation. J Bone Joint Surg 23:481

Benini A (1976) Ischias ohne Bandscheibenvorfall: Die Stenose des lumbalen Wirbelkanals und ihre klinisch-chirurgische Bedeutung. Huber, Bern

Bianco AJ (1968) Low back pain and sciatica: Diagnosis and indication for treatment. J Bone Joint Surg [Am] 50:170–181

Böhni A (1964) Differentialdiagnose der rheumatischen Wirbelsäulenerkrankungen. Rheum Forsch Prax 2:44

Bösch J (1969) Erfahrungen bei 1351 Bandscheibenoperationen aus 21 Jahren. Z Orthop 106:295–301

Brodsky AE (1976) Post-laminectomy and post-fusion stenosis of the lumbar spine. Clin Orthop 115:130–139

Buchmann J (1966) Bemerkungen zur Kokzygodynie. Z Orthop 102:217–231

Campbell RC, Newman PH (1971) Lumbar spondylotomy. J Bone Joint Surg [Br] 53:575–577

De Palma AF, Rothman RH (1969) Surgery of the lumbar spine. Clin Orthop 63:162–170

Ghormley RK (1933) Low back pain with special reference to the articular facts with presentation of an operative procedure. JAMA 101:1773

Gschwend N (1965) Die Bedeutung der Scheuermann'schen Krankheit. Med Hyg 23:612

Hackenbruch W, Hipp E, Gumppenberg S von (1979) Kreuzschmerz. Orthop Prax 15:206–212

Harrington P, Tullos HS (1971) Spondylolisthesis in children. Clin Orthop 79:75–84

Hirsch C, Nachemson A (1963) The reliability of lumbar disc surgery. Clin Orthop 29:191

Hirsch C, Jonsson B, Levin T (1969) Low-back symptoms in a Swedish female population. Clin Orthop 63:171–176

Holt EP (1968) The question of lumbar discography. J Bone Joint Surg [Am] 50:720–726

Krokowski E (1965) Osteoporoseschmerz und Röntgenbefund. Dtsch Med Wochenschr 16:393

Krupp S, Levy A (1963) Zeitliches Zusammentreffen des lumbalen Zwischenwirbelvorfalls mit Schwangerschaft, Geburt und Wochenbett. Geburtshilfe Frauenheilkd 23:130

Kuhlendahl H, Hensell W (1953) Der mediane Massenprolaps der Lendenbandscheiben mit Cauda-Kompression. Dtsch Med Wochenschr 78:332

Lettin AEF (1967) Diagnosis and treatment of lumbar instability. J Bone Joint Surg [Br] 49:520–529

Lindblom K (1948) Diagnostic puncture of intervertebral discs in sciatica, Acta Orthop Scand 17:231

Mensor MC, Duvall G (1959) Absence of motion at the 4th and 5th lumbar interspaces in patients with and without low back pain. J Bone Joint Surg [Am] 41:1047–1054

Macnab I (1977) Backache. Williams & Wilkins, Baltimore

Mixter WJ, Barr JS (1934) Rupture of the intervertebral disc with involvment of the spinal canal. N Engl J Med 211:210

Mooney V, Robertson J (1976) The facet syndrome. Clin Orthop 115:149–156

Morgan FP, King T (1957) Primary instability of lumbar vertebra as a common cause of low back pain. J Bone Joint Surg [Br] 39:6–22

Morscher E (1970) Operative Aufrichtung fixierter Hyperkyphosen durch vordere Wirbelsäulenosteotomie. Z Orthop 108:516–520

Morscher E (1972) Operative Therapie des Kreuzschmerzes. Orthopaede 1:189–201

Morscher E (1975) Zweizeitige Reposition und Stabilisation der Spondyloptose mit dem Harrington-Instrumentarium und vorderer interkorkporeller Spondylodese. Arch Orthop Unfallchir 83:323–334

Morscher E, Figner G (1972) Die Messung der Beinlängen. Orthopaede 1:9–13

Morscher E, Friedrich H (1971) Idiopathic ischemic necrosis of the femoral heads in adults. Thieme, Stuttgart, p 158

Morscher E, Taillard W (1965) Die Beinlängenunterschiede. Karger, Basel

Nachemson A (1960) Lumbar intradiscal pressure. Acta orthop scand suppl 43

Nachemson AL (1971) Low back pain. Its etiology and treatment. Clin Med 78:18–24

Nachemson A (1978) Low Back Pain, Instruct course lecture, 14th congress of Soc internat chir orthop et de traumatol (Sicot), Kyoto/Japan

Newman PH (1963) The etiology of spondylolisthesis. J Bone Joint Surg [Br] 45:39–59

Newman PH (1973) Surgical treatment for derangement of the lumbar spine. J Bone Joint Surg [Br] 55:7–19

Niethard FU, Gaertner B (1979) Der von den kleinen Wirbelgelenken ausgehende Schmerzzustand – das sogenannte Facettensyndrom. Orthop Prax 15:201–203

Pechel E (1965) Die Beckenring-Distorsion und der Symphysenschaden in der Schwangerschaft. Med Heute 14:115

Reinhard H, Heinemann M (1964) Der Aussagewert der Röntgenuntersuchung der Lendenwirbelsäule und der Lumbosakralregion beim Kreuzschmerz der Frau. Med Klin 59:91

Rompe G (1965) Zur Häufigkeitsverteilung röntgenologisch nachweisbarer Strukturunregelmäßigkeiten der Wirbelkörperschlußplatten. Z Orthop 100:16–20

Ross E (1963) Die enchondrale Dysostose der Wirbelsäule. ROEFO 98:578

Schmorl G, Junghanns H (1951) Die gesunde und die kranke Wirbelsäule in Röntgenbild und Klinik, 2nd edn. Thieme Stuttgart

Seidel K, Bertram T (1974) Verbesserung der Indikation gleichzeitiger Dekompression und Fusion durch röntgenologische Objektivierung der lumbalen Instabilitas intervertebralis. Z Orthop 112:867

Severin E (1944) Degeneration of the intervertebral disc in the lumbar region. Acta Chir Scand 89:353

Shealy CN (1976) Facet denervation in the management of back and sciatic pain. Clin Orthop 115:157–164

Sollmann AH (1964) Der Wert der Röntgenkinematographie in der Beurteilung von funktionellen Wirbelsäulenschäden. Wirbelsäule Forsch Prax 28:71–76

Spranger M (1972) Beitrag zur Differentialdiagnose der Veränderungen im Symphysenbereich. Arch Orthop Unfallchir 72:72

Taillard W (1957) Les spondylolisthésis. Masson, Paris

Unander-Scharin L (1950) On low back pain with special reference to the value of operative treatment with fusion. Acta orthop scand suppl 5

Verbiest H (1975) Pathomorphological aspects of developmental lumbar stenosis. Orthop Clin North Am 6:177

Vidal J, Allieu Y, Fassio B, Adrey J, Goalard C (1973) Le spondylolisthésis, réducation par le matérial de Harrington. Rev Chir Orthop 59:21

17 Chronic Pelvic Pain of Urologic Origin (R. L. Vereecken)

17.1 Introduction

There are a number of urologic conditions that may cause chronic pelvic pain. For example, recurrent cystitis and infiltrating bladder tumors provoke pain in the hypogastrium; pain due to an ectopic kidney has a somewhat higher localization, and the pain due to an obstruction of the distal ureter is localized in an iliac fossa and usually radiates to the lumbar region.

Patients suffering acute attacks of pain accompanied by other severe urologic symptoms will be referred to the urologist rather than to the gynecologist. When the complaint is chronic pelvic pain or lower abdominal discomfort, it may create problems that the gastroenterologist, the gynecologist, or the urologist will have to diagnose by a series of appropriate technical investigations. It should be noticed, however, that negative results of an exhaustive exploration may lead to erroneous conclusions. The patient may, indeed, sometimes be mistaken for a neurotic even though there are no positive psychopathologic arguments for this assumption. It should be stressed that so-called psychosomatic symptoms may mask a somatic disease, which for some reason has not been discovered by means of objective investigations. This can be exemplified by a patient who had consulted many doctors for intermittent attacks of pelvic and loin pains. The symptoms remained unexplained for a whole year, after which they were finally explained by the presence of a pediculated tumor just above the vesicoureteral junction. In previous urographies, the polyp had prolapsed into the bladder and had been shielded by thick layers of contrast fluid. Another danger is that some deviations from the normal may be considered causative factors although a causal relationship has never been proved. We will come back to this problem when discussing the right ovarian vein syndrome.

In this chapter, only the most important urologic syndromes that may cause chronic pelvic pain will be surveyed.

17.2 Recurrent Cystourethritis

Neither the diagnosis nor the treatment of acute cystitis is a great problem. Hypogastric pain, dysuria, frequency of micturition, burning, nycturia, urgency accompanied by pyuria, and a positive urine culture are the well-known symptoms, which readily disappear after an adequate antibiotic therapy. Reinfections and relapses are not infrequent. The right antibiotic should be chosen and the duration of therapy adapted; on the other hand, the diagnosis is usually easy.

Asymptomatic bacteriuria falls outside the scope of this book, which deals essentially with pain.

The difficulties start when subjective complaints of cystitis keep recurring although repeated laboratory tests of the urine do not provide an objective confirmation of the diagnosis. In the French literature, this condition is called "cystalgie à urines claires." This syndrome is frustrating for the patient who contracts it because of the inefficiency of the therapies applied and perplexing for the physician who may feel inclined to jump to the conclusion that the patient is a neurotic. Although psychometric tests showed the frequency of anxiety, sexual problems, and other psychiatric disturbances to be three times higher in such patients (Rees 1978), it is unclear whether psychological predispositions were actualized by organic or pathophysiologic disorders or whether the psychological symptoms were merely their results. It should be stressed, indeed, that biopsies of the trigone – a diagnostic technique too often neglected – show a very high percentage of inflammatory cell infiltrates (Rees 1978). It is now recognized that chronic cystitis, with or without sterile urine, is a multifactorial disease and that each etiologic irritative or inflammatory factor may precipitate symptoms, either by itself or in combination with others.

Possible causative factors include the following:

1) Many women hold urine for considerable periods of time; they therefore often reduce fluid intake. This habit has been considered a sign of overcivilization since there are fewer public toilets for women than for men. The bladder suffers from overdistension, resulting in loss of the viscoelastic properties of its wall and in retention of urine. Urinary pathogens, multiplying at an exponential rate, rapidly reach high concentrations. The concentrated urine favors bacterial colonization. Simple reeducation, with scheduled voiding and drinking, will resolve most cases.

2) A variety of affections, such as "urethral syndrome," "female prostatism," "bladder neck tightness," and "épine irritative de l'urèthre" point to the widespread conception of some kind of urethral obstruction as a cause of chronic cystitis complaints. Internal urethrotomies and dilatations of the urethra with all kinds of rubber or metal bougies repeated weekly or monthly are of questionable benefit to the patient's urethra, although we do not deny that such treatment may sometimes give some psychological reassurance and support. In fact, urodynamic assessments prove that bladder outlet obstruction is found in only 10% of these patients (Rees 1978). Bladder trabeculation, seen either at cystoscopy or at cystography, is no longer considered an expression of lower urinary tract obstruction only; it is in fact a sign of bladder instability. This instability may be caused by a variety of sensory and motor factors and is easily detected during cystometry by the presence of uninhibited bladder contractions with amplitudes of more than 15 cm of water.

3) Tanagho et al. (1971) noticed that spasm of the external urethral sphincter, which may lead to hypertrophy, could be a cause of recurrent cystitis. Starting as a conscious reaction during painful urination, the contraction of the pelvic floor musculature during micturition remains as a bad habit in the absence of urinary infection. It impedes a forceful urinary stream that washes out bacteria adherent to the urethral wall and causes a turbulent flow in a dilated proximal urethra ("spinning top"). Reeducation, possibly aided by biofeedback methods (e. g., listening to the EMG signals of the urethral sphincter during voiding, coughing, active contraction, and relaxation) may disrupt the vicious circle.

4) A urethral diverticulum is a well-defined affection that must be cured surgically. Taking into account the numerous periurethral glands, it is astonishing that the affection is not observed more frequently. While the diagnosis is evident in the presence of a fluctuating swelling of the anterior vaginal wall, chronic diverticulitis is often only diagnosed by urethrography with a double-balloon

catheter, with a CO_2 urethroscope of Robertson, or with a permictional and postvoiding urethrography.

5) Recent investigations have clearly demonstrated that nongonococcal urethritis (NGU) is caused by pathogens that can be cultured only in paticular media. Many supposedly sterile urines give positive cultures for *Clamydia,* urea plasmas (T mycoplasma), *Trichomonas, Corynebacterium.* These agents are sexually transmitted, and adequate and simultaneous treatment of both partners is indicated.

6) A careful gynecologic examination is always mandatory since associated or contributory gynecologic factors are present in a high number of women with recurrent cystitis. Rees (1978) listed the gynecologic findings in such patients and noticed a significant percentage of vulvovaginitis and cervical erosions.

The relation between coitus and cystitis is well-documented. "Honey-moon" cystitis may be the start of recurrent cystitis, which may last for several years. The accepted therapy nowadays is precoital vaginal instillation of sulfonamide cream, postcoital voiding, and long-term low-dosage urinary antiseptics or antibiotics (e. g., 1 tablet of nitrofuran or co-trimoxazole daily).

7) Defective toilet hygiene of the perianal region, which may cause fecal contamination, as well as excessive hygiene (with abundant use of bubble baths, vaginal aerosols, bath salts, oils, antiseptics, body lotions, and spermicidal foams), which may cause vulvovaginitis, are predisposing and easily avoidable factors.

8) Interstitial cystitis, also called Hunner ulcer, is still a much discussed subject. Biopsies of the bladder wall show fibrous infiltration of the muscular layers, increase of the 5-hydroxyproline content, and depositions of complement and IgM. There is increasing evidence of an autoimmune disease. Imperious urge occurs at a bladder expansion of 100–150 ml, above which heavy bladder pain and hematuria occur. Coagulation, instillation of dimethyl sulfoxide or sodium hypochlorite solution, and bladder distension have been proposed, but this uncommon condition will often necessitate an intestinocystoplasty.

17.3 Intractable Suprapubic Pain Due to Infiltrating Bladder Tumors

Twenty-five years ago, Darget and Ballenger (1954) described several techniques of treating intolerable pelvic pain: anesthetic infiltrations or surgical sections of the cauda equina, resection of the superior hypogastric plexus, resection of the hypogastric ganglia or nerves, and section of the pudendal or pelvic splanchnic nerves. At that time, the main indications for some of these exceptional therapies were resistant tuberculosis or aspecific infections. Nowadays, nearly all severe chronic suprapubic (and perineal) pain cases are due to infiltrating carcinomatous tumors of bladder, cervix, and uterus or rectum. Even after irradiation or other treatment, the pain may persist, either as a consequence of the primary disease or as a complication of the treatment itself (e. g., radiation cystitis). Despite a large arsenal of drugs, infiltration of ganglia and nerves is still preferable for patients who require high doses of analgesics. Electric cord stimulation may become an alternative in the future.

17.4 Pelvic Kidney Ectopia

A sacral kidney is a congenital malformation due to incomplctc ascension and rotation of the metanephros during fetal life. The kidney is felt as a mass in front of the promontory, sometimes showing rhythmic displacements due to the pulsations of the great pelvic blood vessels. Although the abnormality may remain symptomless, some patients have, in certain body positions, complaints of pelvic tenderness or heaviness, mostly due either to traction on the vascular pedicles or to compression of presacral nerve plexuses. An ectopic kidney may give problems during pregnancy and during gynecologic operations. Ectopic kidneys are predisposed to obstruction and infection; the pain of hydronephrosis or pyelonephritis is then not located in the loin, but around the umbilicus or in the pelvis. Such complications may require surgery, which will often be delicate because of the multiple small vessels running into the ectopic kidney.

17.5 Nephroptosis

An ectopic kidney must be well-distinguished from nephroptosis (or a wandering kidney), a condition in which the renal artery arises from the lumbar aorta at its normal site. For that reason, tenderness if present always has a component in the loin. Right nephroptosis, with or without lateral rotation of the kidney when the patient is in the upright position, is frequently observed in women; when it occurs on the left side, a tumor of the adrenal or of the upper pole of the kidney must be excluded. Too many nephropexies have been performed with bad results as far as the patients' subjective complaints are concerned; moreover, they have sometimes been complicated by osteitis of the ribs. Before deciding on nephropexy, it must be clearly demonstrated by intravenous urographies taken in the upright position and after furosemide injection that the complaints or the urinary infections are due to intermittent hydronephrosis. Effective control of the symptoms by a Glenard corset it a good preoperative test. The movements of the kidney in nephroptosis may cause small tears eliciting fibromuscular dysplasia of the artery, which in turn may cause hypertension; such a constellation is an imperative indication for surgery.

17.6 Ureteral Causes of Pelvic Pain

Lower quadrant pain radiating to the lumbar region during attacks of pyelonephritis is often caused by anatomic or functional obstructions of the ureter. These may be congenital or acquired.

17.6.1 Congenital Ureteral Obstructions

Congenital urologic abnormalities, especially renal and urethral *duplication* and reflux, are more frequent in girls than in boys. Usually, the affection becomes manifest during childhood by acute pyelonephritic attacks with high fever and pyuria. However, incomplete duplications (Y bifidity with a short common branch) or blind-ending ureteral stumps may remain symptomless until adult life; chronic atypical pain may then be evoked by ureteral hyperpressure due to refluxing urine or antiperistalsis. Surgery may be indicated. Functional *stenosis of the vesicoureteral junction* is another congenital anomaly that often causes vague unilateral flank and abdominal pain in the 3rd or 4th decade of life. The condition is sometimes called "achalasia," referring to an erroneous assimilation with Hirschsprung's disease, a neuromuscular deficiency of the rectum; in fact, the pathologic findings are either an interruption of the muscular layers by collagenous tissue or an excess of circular muscle fibers. Radiocinematography clearly shows the dilated distal third of the ureter exhibiting vigorous contractions, which cause variable amounts of urine to reflux to the kidney pelvis. Since the renal function and the clumsy configuration of the calyces may remain stable for many years, a wait-and-see policy is advisable.

17.6.2 Acquired Ureteral Obstructions

Acquired ureteral obstructions causing lower quadrant pelvic pain include periosteal bladder tumors, incomplete obstructions by stones in the distal ureter, infection or dilatation of ureteral stumps left after nephrectomy (performed mainly to treat tuberculosis or reflux), iatrogenic reflux (e. g., after stone extractions), endometriosis of the ureter, and right ovarian vein syndrome. We will limit our discussion to these last two conditions.

17.6.2.1 Endometriosis of the Ureter

The urinary tract is involved in only 1% of all patients with endometriosis: the usual localization is the trigone, but the pelvic ureter may also be affected while the proximal ureter never is. Two forms exist: in the extrinsic type, the ureter is surrounded by a sheath of fibrous tissue caused by endometriotic lesions; in the intrinsic type, foci of endometriosis are found in the lamina propria and muscular layer of the ureter, giving the aspect of a tumor. Although the latter variety may produce a pathognomonic cyclic hematuria, the most common complaints are those due to obstructions, often with cyclic exacerbations. In the absence of obstruction, hormonal treatment may be tried (see Chap. 11). Usually, the periureteral fibrosis requires a resection of the ureter with ureterocystoneostomy. Early detection is necessary to preserve the renal function; fortunately, the history of the urinary symptoms is often very short.

17.6.2.2 Ovarian Vein Syndrome

In 1964 Clark described a condition with the following characteristics: right flank pain or discomfort, often occurring premenstrually, dilatation of the ureter proximal to the pelvic brim at 14 cm above the vesicoureteral junction, sometimes recurrent urinary infections, and tortuosity of the ovarian veins on phlebography or surgical exploration. He found the condition only on the right side and near the end of, or after, pregnancy. Until now, about 300 cases have been published, including several in children and nulliparas, and also cases of bilateral or left-sided syndromes.

This puzzling condition evokes two questions: (1) is the venous dilatation a pathologic condition and (2) can the dilated veins cause ureteral obstruction?

Pelvic varicosities of the at uterine and the ovarian venous plexuses are not uncommon. Tubo-ovarian varicocele was described by Ricket as early as 1857. The symptomatology is said to include pain and heaviness in the pelvis, particularly after prolonged standing, backache, dysmenorrhea, dyspareunia, and even unstable bladder symptoms. The so-called pelvic congestion syndrome described by Taylor (1949) is said to be a preliminary stage of pelvic varicosities. Chidekel et al. (1968) found that pelvic varicosities were always present if, on selective left renal phlebography, an ovarian vein was wider than 6 mm and contrast-filled in a retrograde direction down to the level of S-1. In this investigation, the width of the vein and the frequency of incompetent valves were significantly greater in multiparas than in nulliparas, and the authors found the valves to be incompetent in about 40% of the cases examined. Pelvic vein varicosities are thus not an exception. The problem of whether those varicosities may be responsible for pain complaints is discussed in Chap. 18 and in a review article by Renaer et al. (to be published).

On the other hand, it is a common finding that blood vessels make indentations in the contrast-filled ureter; polar vessels may do so at the pyeloureteral junction, the right ovarian vein where it crosses the ureter at L3–4 and the iliac vessels at the pelvic brim. It is also frequently observed, particularly at low diuresis rates, that urine (or contrast fluid) is held up exactly at these places, making spindles or fluid pools. Differences of ureteral caliber between upper and lower ureteral segments are very often observed in urographies of men and women who have no complaints. It should not be forgotten that roentgenograms are only snapshots of a continuous process. Dilatation, especially of the right ureter above the linea innominata, occurs during pregnancy in three-fourths of the patients; direct compression by the enlarged uterus, hypotonicity due to hormonal factors, and sometimes paralysis by infectious agents are sufficient explanations for this phenomenon. Furthermore, a careful look at the published roentgenograms and the case reports on the ovarian vein syndrome reveals two interesting points. First, the level of interruption of the contrast column is variable from the pelvic brim to L-3, and sometimes a contrast pool is seen between these two levels. This seems to imply that many variations or aberrant collaterals or anastomoses of the right ovarian veins must exist, but this has not been varified by the autopsy studies of Duré-Smith (1979). Secondly, most published urographies show concave calyces and a thick renal parenchyma, and no mention is made of late visualization or delayed emptying of the pyelocalyceal systems. Ureteral dilatation does not necessarily mean obstruction, and it is doubtful whether obstruction really existed in most of the published cases. Some pressure studies in the ureter have been done during and after pregnancy, but not in ovarian vein syndrome. Mortensen and Djurhuus (1976) did report a case with intermittent antiperistalsis, but the EMG showed that the retrograde waves started distally in the nondilated pelvic ureteral segment. So far, it has not been

possible to produce ureteral obstruction by experimental dilatation of ovarian veins either in monkeys or in dogs. For years we have followed several cases that could have been considered ovarian vein syndromes, and none of them has shown any deterioration of renal function despite surgical abstinence.
Besides, it is not evident how the ovarian vein could obstruct the ureter. Some authors have described a common connective sheath for both structures, a finding not confirmed by others. Even then, some kind of sclerotic reaction must be present; in that case, the condition would better be considered retroperitoneal fibrosis, which in the idiopathic type also starts from the L-3 level downward, and in the secondary type may be caused by the retroperitoneal spread of an infection from the appendix, the salpinx, or other neighboring structures. Postpartum ovarian vein thrombophlebitis should be considered a separate entity.
All the foregoing facts and considerations leave the present author sceptical about the existence of an ovarian vein syndrome as a cause of chronic iliac fossa pain. As to the reported successes after surgical ligation or resection of ovarian veins, surely not all of them have been unqualified successes and, unfortunately, the duration of follow-up is frequently not reported. On the other hand, this author has had to care for three disasters after such an operation. He feels that one should be very cautious before embarking on the surgical treatment of a condition whose pathogenic influence has not yet been clearly proved.

References

Chidekel N (1968) Female pelvic veins demonstrated by selective renal phlebography with particular reference to pelvic varicosities. Acta Radiol 7, 193

Clark JC (1964) The right ovarian vein syndrome. In: Emmett JL (ed) Clinical urography, 2nd edn. Saunders, Philadelphia, pp 1227–1237

Darget R, Ballanger R (1954) Cystites invétérées et algies pelviennes. Masson, Paris, p 118

Duré-Smith P (1979) Ovarian vein syndrome: is it a myth? Urology 12:355–364

Kremling H (1977) Endometriose. In: Kremling H, Lutzeyer W, Heintz S (eds) Gynäkologische Urologie und Nephrologie. Urban & Schwarzenberg, München, pp 252–253

Mortensen SO, Djurhuus JC (1976) Right ovarian vein syndrome. A case with pre- and peroperative electromyographic registration of ureteral activity. Acta Chir Scand 472:91–93

Rees DLP (1978) Urinary tract infection. Clin Obstet Gynecol 5:169–192

Renaer M, Nijs P, van Assche A, Vertommen H (to be published) Chronic pelvic pain without obvious pathology. Personal observations with a review of the literature. Eur J Obstet Gynecol

Ricket MA (1857) Traité pratique d'anatomie médico-chirurgicale. F Chamerot, Libraire Editeur, Paris

Tanagho EA, Miller ER, Lyon RP, Fisher R (1971) Spastic striated external sphincter and urinary tract infection in girls. Br J Urol 43:69–81

Taylor HC (1954) Pelvic pain based on a vascular and autonomic nervous system disorder. Am J Obstet Gynecol 67/2, 1177

18 Chronic Pelvic Pain Without Obvious Pathology

18.1 Introduction

Besides the pain syndromes described so far, there are complaints of chronic pelvic pain that are apparently of gynecologic origin but for which no definite lesion or cause is found. This syndrome has been known since the first half of the nineteenth century and, depending on the different authors' views concerning its pathogenesis, has been described under many different names.

During the last decades, it has been called the "syndrome of pelvic congestion and fibrosis" (Taylor 1949a, b, c), "pelipathia vegetativa" (Gauss 1949), "pelvic sympathetic syndrome" (Theobald 1951), and "pelvic neurodystonia" (Schockaert 1956).

Several authors deny the existence of this syndrome. Atlee (1966) discards it as "diagnostic garbage." Novak and Jones (1970) find it difficult to believe that there is such a thing as the "so-called generalized pelvic congestion phenomenon." Jeffcoate (1975) admits that there are cases of pelvic congestion, calling them "congestive dysmenorrhea" and ascribing the pain to premenstrual engorgement of the pelvic tissues, but he does not believe in the existence of a condition that was called "broad ligament neuritis" by Young (1938) and "spastic posterior parametritis" under the influence of the German literature.

We feel that the syndrome under discussion is most accurately described by the term chronic pelvic pain without obvious pathology (CPPWOP). To prove that such a syndrome exists in its own right, it has to be shown that:

1) The patient's condition is not due to a nongynecologic cause
2) The pain has the characteristics of a pain of gynecologic origin
3) The syndrome is not due to one of the acknowledged causes of gynecologic pain
4) No definite lesion has been found

The differential diagnosis between gynecologic and nongynecologic causes of pelvic pain has been dealt with in several other chapters. The various acknowledged causes of pelvic pain of gynecologic origin have also been described. The absence of organic lesions has to be demonstrated by careful clinical, laparoscopic, and sometimes hysterographic investigation.

We believe that a limited number of patients fulfill the four conditions just mentioned (Renaer et al. 1980).

18.2 Description of the Syndrome

The most important symptom is lower abdominal pain and, less frequently, low back pain. The lower abdominal pain may be felt either in the whole lower abdomen, in both iliac fossae, or in one fossa only. The low back pain may be felt over the whole width of the sacrogluteal zone or over one-half of this zone only.

The pain is usually more severe for several days before the menses and abates on the 1st or 2nd day of the period, although continuous pain is by no means exceptional. It usually increases when the patient has been standing upright for some time and also when she runs, jumps, or sits down brusquely. It is alleviated by horizontal rest. Deep dyspareunia is a frequent complaint.

Besides the pain symptoms, other complaints, such as leukorrhea, menstrual disturbances, constipation, cystalgia, asthenia, depression, and anxiety are mentioned with variable frequency, depending on the authors. The present writer would, however, not consider leukorrhea, menstrual disturbances, constipation, or cystalgia to be common symptoms of the syndrome.

Most patients are married, and the symptoms frequently start a short time after a delivery. The syndrome is most often seen between 20 and 40 years of age, seldom in the climacteric and never after menopause.

On gynecologic examination, the uterus and adnexa may be tender; marked tenderness of the posterior parametrium is also a frequent finding. Some authors state that a cervicitis may be found; we prefer to exclude the cases with cervicitis because a chronic cervicitis coinciding with the presence of a tender posterior parametrium is probably a different syndrome, which we have termed "posterior parametritis due to a chronic cervicitis" in Chap. 12.

When a chronic pelvic pain syndrome has lasted for several months and has not been relieved by medical treatment, it is indicated to perform a laparoscopy to look for nonpalpable lesions, such as endometriosis or sequelae of chronic PID, which might explain the pain. By definition, those lesions are not found in CPPWOP; in fact, the presence of a CPPWOP syndrome should only be admitted when all examinations, including laparoscopy, have failed to reveal any acknowledged cause of chronic pelvic pain. In the CPPWOP syndrome, two varieties or clinical forms can be distinguished.

The first variety seems to be the least frequent. The pain has a symmetric localization in the lower abdomen; it is most pronounced during the premenstrual period and tends to disappear on the 1st day of menstruation. The uterus and adnexa are tender on palpation, and there may or may not be tenderness of the sacrouterine ligaments or the posterior parametrium. Some authors stress that inspection of the cervix reveals a cyanotic cervical mucosa. Some patients have a similar pain syndrome lasting several days in the paraovulatory period; in these instances, the syndrome could also be considered a prolonged episode of mittelschmerz. The symptoms of this first variety are suggestive of circulatory disturbances.

In the second form, the pain may have either a symmetric or unilateral localization; it does not always disappear during menstruation, and on gynecologic examination, there is always tenderness of the posterior parametrium. Frequently, there are painful anteroposterior condensations or densifications in the parameterium, and sometimes the posterior parametrium is shortened so that the cervix is found in retroposition. When pressure or traction is exerted on the sacrouterine ligaments, this maneuver generally reproduces the spontaneous pain and the deep dyspareunia.

18.3 Prevalence

As can be seen Table 1 (Chap. 1), CPPWOP was found in 28 of a series of 108 patients who had been taken into the clinic for a complete work-up and whose main complaint was chronic pelvic pain.

18.4 Pathogenesis

The pathogenesis of this syndrome has been a matter of debate for many years now. It is important both from a theoretical and from a practical point of view because over the years the divergent opinions expressed have led to equally diverse therapeutic solutions.

In a recent paper, we have confronted the literature on the subject published during the last decades with our own observations (Renaer et al. 1980). We will therefore repeatedly refer to this review.

Before considering the various possible pathogenetic mechanisms, it is worthwile to give a few details of the clinical history and the examination of 31 patients with CPPWOP who were carefully observed with the express view of testing several recent pathogenetic theories.

In those 31 patients, the pain was localized either in the lower abdomen or in the lower abdomen and in the sacrogluteal zone. It was either symmetric or unilateral. Seventeen patients complained of deep dyspareunia.

In 12 cases, there were several complaints, including one or more that are generally considered "functional," such as headache, asthenia, palpitations, nausea, epigastric discomfort, irritability, and depression; these patients may be called polysymptomatic. Most oligosymptomatic patients merely complained of spontaneous pain and deep dyspareunia.

Palpation almost never revealed an oversized or tender uterus, as described in some papers. The volume of the cervix was seldom augmented and it only rarely had a cyanotic appearance. However, uni- or bilateral tenderness of the sacrouterine ligaments or the posterior parametrium was found frequently. In a few cases, this tenderness was accompanied by shortening of the posterior parametrium and densifications in the anteroposterior direction. There were no cases of retroversion among the 31 patients. All had undergone a laparoscopy because no case should be classified as CPPWOP unless the acknowledged pain-provoking pelvic lesions have been excluded by careful gynecologic examination and endoscopic verification.

During the last decades, the following conditions have been suspected as possible causes of CPPWOP: (1) traumatic laceration of the supporting structures of the uterus (Allen and Masters 1955), (2) circulatory disturbances, (3) structural or functional modifications of the sacrouterine ligaments, and (4) psychogenic mechanisms. We will briefly analyze the evidence for and against the possible influence of these factors.

18.4.1 To What Extent Is CPPWOP Due to "Traumatic Laceration of Uterine Support"?

In Allen and Masters' paper on "Traumatic Laceration of Uterine Support" (1955), the most common complaints are dyspareunia (24 of 28 cases), excessive physical fatigue (24/28), dysmenorrhea (22/28), and generalized pelvic distress (21/28). The majority of the patients were polysymptomatic and presented complaints of a functional nature.

Table 9 shows the pelvic pathologic changes found in the 28 cases of Allen and Masters (1955). As stated in Table 9, all 28 cases had a third-degree retroversion, and it was noted that "the uterus was increased, was soft, and had the purplish red cast so frequently noted in hemostasis, and it shrank in size when it was brought forward."

In all cases, the laceration was repaired; in 23 cases, a Gilliam's suspension operation was performed, and in the 5 remaining cases the uterus was later found in anteversion even though no suspension operation had been done. It is therefore difficult to know whether the disappearance of the complaints was due to the repair of the laceration or to the reduction of the retroversion.

Truc and Musset (1973) give an extensive review of the syndrome. The papers they quote are essentially of French origin; indeed, the syndrome seems to be less frequently diagnosed in Germany and seldom in the United States and Great Britain. Even in France, the frequency with which the syndrome is diagnosed differs greatly from one center to another. Whereas in some centers, 108 (Keller et al. 1972) or 132 cases (Serment 1972 cited by Truc and Musset 1973) have been operated on, Palmer (1973 cited by Truc and Musset 1973) found it only 3 times in 400 laparoscopies performed for pain. In a diligent 12-year search, Truc and Musset (1973) found only ten cases, four of whom they operated on. In more than 1000 laparoscopies, several hundreds of which were done for chronic lower abdominal pain, we only once saw what may have been a real tear in a sacrouterine ligament.

The drawings in the paper by Allen and Masters (1955) show a tear of the posterior leaf of a broad ligament and one in a broad ligament and a sacrouterine ligament. However, in publications by others, the lesion is not really a

Table 9. Pelvic pathology in 28 cases. Allen and Masters (1955) Traumatic laceration of uterine support. Am J Obs Gyn 70:500–513

Pathology demonstrated	Total cases with positive report
Third-degree retroversion of the uterus	28
Serous fluid in the pelvis (30–80 ml)	27
Bilateral broad ligament laceration	22
Unilateral broad ligament laceration	6
Unilateral sacrouterine ligament laceration	5
Bilateral sacrouterine ligament laceration	1

tear but a depression of the posterior leaf of the broad ligament, in the depth of which depression varicose veins are frequently reported. The divergence in the prevalence of the syndrome may therefore be due to the fact that the name "Allen and Masters' syndrome" is given to different pathologic conditions.
We believe that real tears in the supporting structures of the uterus are very rare; our recent observations (Renaer et al. 1980) could not convince us of a causal relationship between chronic pelvic pain and a depression in a posterior leaf of a broad ligament or in the peritoneal covering of a sacrouterine ligament.
We therefore feel that the role of the Allen and Masters' syndrome in the explanation of CPPWOP is negligible, and we wonder whether the symptoms found in most cases described in the literature were not due to painful mobile retroversion. Even so, it is astonishing that so many cases of painful retroversion are found in some centers, whereas most gynecologists rarely see any.

18.4.2 Role of Circulatory Disturbances in the Pathogenesis of CPPWOP

It is plausible that circulatory factors can provoke pain in the female internal genital organs. The circulatory anomaly may be either active or passive hyperemia.
The first modifications observed in the uterine wall of castrated female animals after the administration of estrogens is an increase in blood flow and retained water (Reynolds 1949; Greiss and Anderson 1970; Makowski 1977). The lower abdominal pain some postmenopausal women experience a few days after the beginning of an estrogen treatment can probably be explained by an increased intratissular pressure in the uterine wall, resulting from a sharp increase in blood flow. The same mechanism apparently explains some cases of prolonged mittelschmerz whose duration seems to coincide with the paraovulatory estrogen peak; these cases may also be due to the increased basal tone of the uterine contractions during this period (Hein et al. 1972). It should be noted, however, that increased blood flow can hardly be the sole explanation of the pain as lower abdominal pain is rarely found in the beginning of pregnancy, where we must assume that there is an important rise in the myometrial blood flow (Makowski 1977).
Several authors (Cotte 1949; Taylor 1949 a, b, c; Jeffcoate 1975) believe that in some patients lower abdominal pain may be due to increased intramural pressure caused by passive congestion during the premenstrual period. The French call this "pelvic congestion" and the English "congestive dysmenorrhea."
Passive or venous congestion is, in our opinion, the most probable cause of the pain in cases of painful mobile retroversion, which is uncommon (see Chap. 6). In these cases, the size of the uterus is frequently increased, the uterus is soft and tender on palpation, and it becomes firmer and less tender with the disappearance of the spontaneous pain, within 2 or 3 days after replacement of the retroversion. It is the uterine corpus rather than the posterior parametrium that is tender in cases of painful mobile retroversion, whereas the reverse is observed in most cases of CPPWOP. The fact that CPPWOP is almost never seen after menopause also favors a circulatory explanation of the pain.

As long as we cannot perform sufficiently exact measurements of uterine blood flow, we will be unable to prove to what extent circulatory anomalies play a role in the pathogenesis of CPPWOP. This means that at the moment the problem can only be approached by indirect methods; this has been done by means of uterine phlebography and laparoscopy.
In our more extensive study, we concluded our review of the literature on phlebography in chronic pelvic pain syndromes as follows:

> ... a good many of the patients with CPPWOP present radiological signs of passive pelvic congestion, but a certain percentage do not present those signs. On the other hand, persons who do not complain of pain may also have radiological signs of passive pelvic congestion and therefore, other factors besides passive pelvic congestion must intervene te explain the pain.

Several authors have emphasized that in patients with "pelvic congestion" a great amount of straw-colored fluid is usually found in the pelvis, and this "increased transudation" is taken as another indirect argument for the presence of venous stasis.
In a comparative study, we performed a laparoscopy on 16 patients with CPPWOP, on 16 patients whose pain was most probably due to endometriosis, and on 15 patients who did not complain of pain but had to undergo a laparoscopy for the evaluation of their infertility. In all those patients, we looked for the presence of a large "mottled" uterus, for the presence or absence of varicosities in the infundibulopelvic ligaments and in the uterine veins at the basis of the broad ligament, and we aspirated and measured the fluid found in the pouch of Douglas (Koninckx et al. 1980).
In none of the 16 patients with CPPWOP did we see a strikingly enlarged uterus. A mottled appearance of the uterus was found only once, but this may also occasionally be seen in patients who do not complain of pain. As most of our patients with CPPWOP were on contraceptive steroids at the time of the laparoscopy, we had to resort to yet another control series of patients who did not complain of pain, who where on contraceptive steroids, and who were of comparable parity. There was no striking difference in the frequency of varices between the two series of patients.
Maathuis et al. (1978) and Koninckx et al. (1980) have shown that the amount of peritoneal fluid found during the normal menstrual cycle is quite variable. This variability seems essentially due to hormonally determined changes in vascular permeability, leading to a change of the equilibrium between inflow and outflow across the peritoneal membrane and, to some extent, to fluid transfer at the level of the ovarian surface after and possibly before follicular rupture (Maathuis et al. 1978). The presence of pelvic varices does not influence the amount of peritoneal fluid (Koninckx et al. 1980).
Although we have not had the opportunity to compare the volume of peritoneal fluid in a series of patients with CPPWOP with normal menstrual cycles and a comparable series of patients without pain, we believe that it remains to be demonstrated that a greater amount of peritoneal fluid is found in patients with CPPWOP.
In conclusion, there is good circumstantial evidence that circulatory factors may give rise to chronic or intermittent lower abdominal pain. There is phlebo-

graphic evidence for the presence of passive pelvic congestion in a percentage of cases with CPPWOP, but this passive pelvic congestion is not the sole factor at work in causing the pain. A clear-cut demonstration of the importance of circulatory factors in the genesis of the pain will have to await better methods for the evaluation of pelvic circulation. From a practical point of view, it follows that the presence of indirect signs pointing toward pelvic congestion should not too easily lead to surgical operations, such as suspension procedures, ligature of varicosities, or hysterectomy.

18.4.3 To What Extent Can the Syndrome Be Explained by Morphological or Functional Modifications in the Internal Genital Organs or in the Parametrium?

Taylor (1949a, b, c) found the uterus enlarged in 32 of his 105 cases of "pelvic congestion." In describing the clinical findings in cases of "pelvic congestion syndrome," Montgomery (1966) and Parsons and Sommers (1978) stated that the fundus is frequently felt in retroversion and seems soft, "boggy," and definitely enlarged. Although painful mobile retroversion seems to be a good example of pelvic congestion, we prefer not to include such cases in the discussion of CPPWOP to concentrate on factors that are not related to the retroversion. In the majority of our cases, the uterus was normal in size, and we do not know of any study showing specific morphological changes in the uterine corpus in cases of CPPWOP.

For years, many French authors have considered the so-called sclerocystic dystrophy of the ovaries a rather frequent cause of pelvic pain. In our own series of 31 cases, we did not find a single one in which the ovaries presented an anomaly that could be considered the cause of the pain.

Most authors who have studied CPPWOP stress that they frequently found tenderness of the uterosacral ligaments or of the posterior parametrium. The names found in the German literature to designate the syndrome [parametritis posterior chronica, parametritis posterior (Freund 1903; Freund 1933; Martin 1944), and parametropathia spastica (Martius 1939)] bear witness to this fact. Taylor (1949a, b, c) states that the single most characteristic sign of "pelvic congestion" is tenderness of the uterosacral ligaments; this sign was present in 98 of 105 of his patients.

In the earlier German literature, this tenderness was thought to be due an inflammatory process, but since the reports by Opitz (1922), Louros (1927), Neumann (1933), and Martius (1939), the tenderness has generally been ascribed to a spastic contraction of the smooth muscle fibers of the paracervical tissue. According to Knörr et al. (1972), the "spasm" of the ligaments disappears under anesthesia, and according to Prill (1964), it yields under the influence of relaxation and reassurance.

Histologic studies performed on superior hypogastric plexuses (Cotte and Dechaume 1931), on the uterosacral ligaments (Neumann 1933), on parametrial tissue (Laszlo and Györy 1959, 1963), and on the pelvic peritoneum (De Brux et al. 1968) have failed to demonstrate any clear-cut characteristic anomaly; unfortunately, all those studies lacked adequate controls.

In our own cases, 26 of 31 presented a striking tenderness of the posterior parametrium when it was stretched during vaginal or rectovaginal examination. In most patients, the pain that is provoked on stretching the posterior parametrium reproduces the pain they experience spontaneously or during intercourse. It must, however, be pointed out that in a minority of our cases no tenderness of the posterior parametrium was found.

The tenderness of the sacrouterine ligaments or of the posterior parametrium does not seem to be due to a spasm of smooth muscle bundles because in most cases there was only tenderness and no shortening and because in those cases in which anteroposterior indurations or condensations were found, no noticeable lengthening of the posterior parametrium and no modification of the consistency of the condensations was found during examination under anesthesia.

In our own laboratory, Van Assche (Renaer et al. 1980) extensively investigated the pathology of the cervix and the posterior parametrium in eight patients with CPPWOP who underwent a hysterectomy for their pain and in six patients without pain who underwent a hysterectomy either for menorrhagia due to fibroids or for metrorrhagia due to dysfunctional bleeding. Van Assche could not find a significant difference between the specimens from the pain cases and those from the controls. Interstitial edema was more pronounced in the cervix and the posterior parametrium in three pain cases; this may, however, have resulted from the fact that these three patients had been taking 5 mg of ethinylestrenol daily for several weeks before surgery. Thus, Van Assche did not find a clear morphological explanation either for the tenderness or for the painful condensations frequently found in the posterior parametrium.

In summary, tenderness with or without shortening of the posterior parametrium is a characteristic finding in the majority of cases of CPPWOP; as pressure or traction exerted on the posterior parametrium usually reproduces the pain the patient feels either spontaneously or during intercourse, this condition seems to intervene in the pain mechanism in many cases of CPPWOP. However, the morphological or functional basis of this tenderness remains to be elucidated; it is not known at present whether it is due to an earlier inflammation or whether it is the result of a prolonged state of pelvic congestion.

Tenderness of the posterior parametrium is not present in all cases of CPPWOP and therefore does not offer a universal explanation of all cases. Furthermore, a painful posterior parametrium does not explain the various other symptoms of many polysymptomatic patients. Finally, the problem remains as to why some patients with a tender posterior parametrium only complain of deep dyspareunia and no spontaneous pain and why some persons with a tender posterior parametrium do not complain at all.

Up to now, no clear-cut organic or pathophysiologic cause has been found for the pain in CPPWOP. On the other hand, many of these patients are polysymptomatic and besides their chronic pelvic pain, have a whole array of diverse "functional" symptoms. This observation has led many authors to examine the psychology of these patients.

18.4.4 Psychological Characteristics of Women with CPPWOP

A critical survey of the recent literature on these psychological characteristics can be found in our review article (Renaer et al. 1980). This survey can be summarized by saying that all the authors found definite psychopathologic anomalies or stress situations in almost all patients examined.
In our own patients we approached this problem in three different ways.

1) We compared the symptoms of 24 patients with CPPWOP with those of 22 patients whose pain was most probably due to endometriosis. Whereas only 1 of 22 patients with pain due to endometriosis had more than four different complaints, 12 of 24 patients with CPPWOP had four complaints or more, and the polysymptomatic patients generally had several complaints that are usually considered "functional," functional being defined here as a complaint that has no clear organic or pathophysiologic basis.
2) The psychopathologic evaluation by our psychiatrists of the above-mentioned 24 patients with CPPWOP showed that several patients exhibited neurotic behavior. These were, on the other hand, many patients who labored under stress situations, which in most cases were antecedent to the complaints. There is unfortunately no control group for this part of our psychological investigations, but according to our psychiatrists, these patients certainly differed as a group from a large series of persons who did not complain of pain and who were seen for an evaluation of their requests for sterilization. We can thus conclude that patients with CPPWOP have a gamut of diverse psychological problems, such as neurotic behavior and difficult physical or psychological life situations.
3) In the third part of our psychological evaluation, we set out to compare quantitatively the psychological characteristics of patients with CPPWOP to those of patients suffering from pain with a known organic basis (Renaer et al. 1979).

A battery of psychometric tests, the Minnesota multiphasic personality inventory (MMPI) of Hathaway and Kinley (1951), the Amsterdam biographical questionnaire (ABVV) of Wilde (1963), and the interpersonal relations questionnaire (VIR) of Vertommen and Rochette (1978), were administered to 15 patients with CPPWOP (group I), to 22 patients with pain due to endometriosis (group II), and to 23 control patients (group III) who did not complain of pain and had been admitted into the clinic for apparently trivial conditions, such as a slight degree of bladder descent or intermenstrual bleeding under contraceptive steroids. Much to our astonishment, statistical analysis showed that groups I and II did not differ significantly on the clinical scales of the MMPI.
Figure 21 clearly shows similar profiles for groups I and II, the two pain groups. The scores of the two pain groups (I and II) clearly indicate a neurotic behavior. About the same holds true for the ABVV.
There is thus no significant difference between the variables concerning the psychic functioning of patients with chronic pain without a clear organic cause and the variables of those with chronic pain of organic origin. These data are in agreement with those of the investigations performed by Bond (1971), Woodforde and Merskey (1972), and Sternbach et al. (1973).

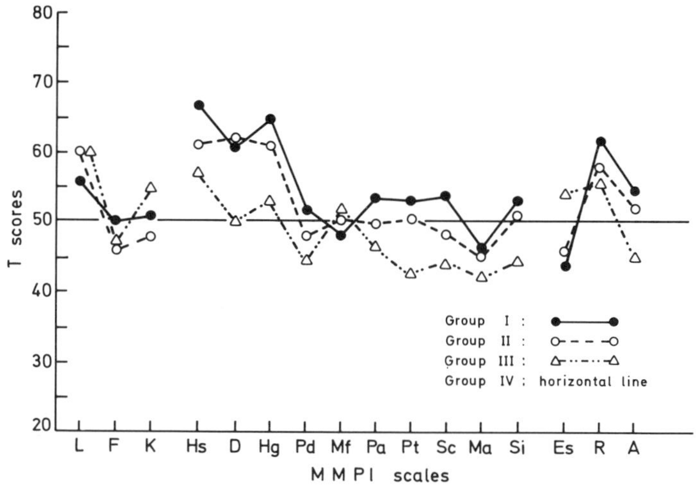

Fig. 21. Means of the groups on the MMPI scales in T values. Renaer M (1979) Psychic aspects of pelvic pain in women. Am G Obs Gyn 134:78

The conclusions of these various papers confirm Sternbach's opinion that although psychometric tests are useful aids in evaluating the patient's personality, "nothing in the battery of pain tests and personality examinations can indicate whether a patient's pain is psychogenic or somatogenic."

In summary, the evaluation of personality and behavior of patients with CPPWOP reveals psychological problems or psychiatric disorders in most of them. According to the psychometric findings of several authors, including our own, this correlation does not allow the conclusion that these psychological problems or disturbances are primary and the pain complaints mere consequences. However, the psychiatric interviews conducted in several series of cases have shown that many patients had a family and personal history that may have induced a maladaptation to the ordinary or extraordinary stresses of their professional or family life. The multifarious functional complaints presented by many patients also point toward important psychogenic influences in the pathogenesis of their complaints. On the other hand, the psychiatric interviews conducted by Prill (1964) and by Nijs and his collaborators on our own patients (Renaer et al. 1980) have shown that some patients' reactions and behavior cannot be considered abnormal.

18.4.5 A Hypothesis Concerning the Pathogenesis of CPPWOP

Because of the absence of obvious pathology on the one hand and the presence in most patients of stress situations and psychopathologic problems on the other, there is an understandable tendency to look for a psychogenic explanation of the syndrome. We should, however, not opt for a simple psychosomatic explanation too readily.

1) The fact that we do not find a satisfactory physical cause does not mean that the cause is psychogenic. There are several examples of conditions that have mistakenly been believed to be due to psychogenic factors, e. g., primary dysmenorrhea. Even if a complaint seems to have an obvious psychogenic origin, we must not jump to conclusions. Fielding (1977) remarks that in the irritable bowel syndrome "it must be anticipated that with increasing knowledge further examples of 'organic' disease will be separated off from the irritable bowel syndrome."
2) Correlation does not mean cause. Rabkin and Struening (1976) have rightly stressed the multifactorial genesis of most cases of chronic illness. Sternbach (1978) draws attention to the complexity of pain experience and expression and emphasizes that "the causative labels psychogenic and somatogenic need not be and frequently are not mutually exclusive."
3) Even when it is probable that a patient's complaints are to a great extent influenced by psychological issues, we still have to explain why she has precisely lower abdominal pain and low back pain and not another pain localization. In the absence of a clear organic cause, this localization may have a psychological origin, e. g., identification with the condition of a friend, or it may be an example of symbolic language. In actual practice, purely psychogenic mechanisms do not seem to explain many cases of chronic pelvic pain. It would therefore seem that the pendulum is swung too far if all cases of CPPWOP are stamped as "mere neurotics."

Besides the cases in whom a meticulous search for a somatogenic cause remains negative and in whom personality and behavior disturbances are found that offer a plausible explanation of the complaint, there are others in whom repeated psychological evaluations by a gynecologist and/or a psychiatrist do not demonstrate any personality disorder or maladaptive behavior. In such cases, it should be admitted that the cause of the pain is most probably organic or pathophysiologic, even though for the time being the pain mechanism is not clear. In between these extremes, there is the patient whose life has been miserable or who is burdened by a stress situation and who makes one wonder which factors, organic or psychologic, are preponderant in the genesis of her complaint.

The explanation of these diverse observations might be that patients with CPPWOP constitute a heterogeneous group, made up of a spectrum of miscellaneous conditions. At one end, there are patients with very little peripheral noxious stimulation and a preponderance of psychogenic factors; in these patients, the complaints will to a large extent have a psychological explanation. The other extreme is made up of persons with rather intense peripheral noxious stimulation – either pelvic circulatory disturbances or tenderness of the posterior parametrium and, more seldom, uterine cramps or a real tear in a sacrouterine ligament – and little or no psychological influences. In between these extremes, there will be a number of mixed cases whose complaints are conditioned by a combination of less pronounced peripheral noxious stimulation and of one or more of the great variety of psychophysiologic mechanisms that may contribute to the complex stimulus constellations that induce complaints and care-seeking behavior (Rabkin and Struening 1976; Chapman 1978; Sternbach 1978).

18.5 Therapeutic Strategy

In view of the complexity of the management of CPPWOP, it is preferable to think in terms of "therapeutic strategy" (Almy 1977) rather than treatment.
To evaluate the results of medical or surgical treatment of chronic pain syndromes, the patient should be followed for at least 1 or 2 years. It is indeed well-known that patients with CPPWOP who undergo an operation may be pleased with the result during the first few months but that after some time they may again start complaining of the same or other symptoms.

18.5.1 Establishing an Efficient Therapeutic Relationship

Even if the physician does not find a satisfactory explanation, the patient's complaint should be taken seriously. The physician should not traumatize her by saying or intimating that it is all "just nerves" or frighten and discourage her by stating that she has an inflammation of the ovaries or varices or a tear, which will have to be operated upon "because they rarely disappear without an operation." Time should be taken to listen to the patient's description of her symptoms and her problems. Most patients have already consulted one or more physicians. It will be useful to see these patients more than once to verify whether the symptoms remain the same or vary.
The doctor should try to obtain information concerning the patient's family and personal history, her marital life, and her general behavior. Inquiries should also be made about the diagnosis formulated and the treatment proposed or performed by other doctors.
Any nongynecologic or any organic gynecologic disorder that could explain the symptoms should be excluded. If a conservative medical treatment prescribed on a probability diagnosis has remained unsuccessful, laparoscopy should be performed to establish a correct diagnosis and to alleviate the anxiety of the patient more efficiently. This diagnostic exploration sometimes suffices to reassure the patient and to raise her "complaining threshold." However, "the reassurance that cancer or other serious diseases are not present has a short half-life" (Almy 1977).
This multiphasic diagnostic exploration will help to discover the problems, the personality, and the reactions of the patient and to locate her on the spectrum of possibilities between a purely psychogenic syndrome and one that seems to have a definite, albeit temporarily unclear, pathophysiologic explanation.

18.5.2 Psychological Evaluation and Treatment

As CPPWOP is frequently associated with psychological problems or with personality disorders, it is important to examine the relationship between psychological factors and the pain complaints; this may sometimes be easy but most often is not. In 2 of the 24 patients referred to in Sect. 18.4.4 the pain disappeared, and in a third patient it became more bearable after the laparoscopy had confirmed the absence of lesions. It is probable that in those cases the pain experience was to a large extent conditioned by anxiety. In yet another patient, the pain seemed to be due to an identification with a friend who had died of cancer after having suffered from chronic lower abdominal pain. There is abundant evidence that pain complaints may be closely related with psychiatric illness (see Chap. 5; Merskey and Spear 1967; Merskey 1978; Pilowsky 1978); they are most frequently associated with depression or anxiety. Pain is often used as a hysterical conversion symptom; it may also be a manifestation of hypochondriasis. Whenever such an association is probable, treatment should address itself to the psychiatric condition. The gynecologist may attempt to do this or may refer the patient to a psychiatrist. Such a referral should, however, not be resorted to too readily because it may result in a breach of the therapeutic relationship between the patient and the gynecologist. When a referral is deemed necessary, it is in the best interest of the patient that a close collaboration be maintained between the gynecologist and the psychiatrist.

18.5.3 Medical Treatment

Signs of cervical infection should be treated with systemic antibiotics. If there is, at the same time, a tender posterior parametrium, there is a possibility that the diagnosis is not CPPWOP in the strict sense, but a posterior parametritis due to cervicitis; local heat in the form of hot sitz baths or diathermy will frequently be useful.

Some patients have been helped with cyclic estroprogestogens; others by a hypoestrogenic amenorrhea induced by continuous administration of progestogens, for example, 5 mg of lynestrenol daily or 5 mg of norethisterone acetate daily during several months. If the pain disappears under continuous progestogen treatment, a reduction of the daily dose to 2.5 mg may be attempted to lessen the anabolic effects of the drug.

If the spontaneous pain disappears under estroprogestogens or progestogens, deep dyspareunia may persist, especially in those cases that have a tender posterior parametrium; it will frequently be alleviated by avoidance of deep penetration during intercourse (see Chap. 14).

Several German and some Anglo-Saxon authors (Young 1947) have used infiltrations of the uterosacral ligaments, either with a local anesthetic or with a depot anesthetic, to block the inferior hypogastric plexus or the hypogastric nerves. We once did use this treatment on many patients but have abandoned it as infiltration of the tender tissues is painful and usually results in only short-lived disappearance of the pain.

18.5.4 Surgical Treatment

Although a priori surgical interruption of the pain-conducting nerve tracts would seem logical, few gynecologists have obtained lasting results either with the resection of the superior hypogastric plexus (Cotte's operation, 1931) or with the transection of the uterosacral liagments to interrupt the hypogastric nerves (Doyle 1955).

Having hardly ever seen a true tear in a uterosacral or broad ligament, we have only once performed a suture of a "depression" in a posterior leaf of a broad ligament, with poor results.

We have never ligated any varicosities of the infundibulopelvic ligaments or of the uterine veins. Several gynecologists who have used this conservative sort of operation have been less than pleased with the results and have stopped performing it (personal communication E. De Muylder, Brussels, and H. Frangenheim, Konstanz).

Wedge resections of so-called sclerocystic ovaries seldom relieve chronic lower abdominal pain; this procedure is frequently followed by recurrence of the pain, and subsequent scars and adhesions reduce the fertility chances of the patient.

In cases of CPPWOP with unilateral pain localization, a salpingo-oophorectomy will only rarely be efficient.

Many gynecologists have performed, and still perform, total hysterectomies for CPPWOP. Taylor (1961) did a hysterectomy in 9 of 114 cases and obtained good results in all of them; he stressed that this operation should not be resorted to unless several conditions have been fulfilled before. According to Mills (1978), a hysterectomy can be strongly recommended in severe cases of CPPWOP; it gives "immediate, dramatic and persistent relief." In former years, before the era of contraceptive pills and oral progestogens, we performed many hysterectomies for chronic lower abdominal pain, only to become discouraged by the rather low percentage of persistent good results. As many others, we have progressively become more reluctant to perform hysterectomies in these cases, and at present, we only resort to a total – never a subtotal – hysterectomy under the following conditions:

- The patient should have completed her family
- She should have been treated conservatively for several months or years
- She should be oligosymptomatic
- No reservations should have been formulated by our psychiatrists

Conclusions about the results of the operation ought to be drawn only after long-term follow-up. Compared with the results we used to obtain when we performed hysterectomies much more readily, we are rather pleased with the results of our conservative management. Of the 24 patients referred to in Sect. 18.4.4, 13 responded well to conservative medical therapy. Six kept complaining, but their symptoms seemed essentially conditioned by psychopathologic disturbances, and it is quite probable that hysterectomy would not have cured them. Three patients underwent a hysterectomy; two of them are feeling better and one still has the same symptoms as before.

References

Allen WM, Masters WH (1955) Traumatic laceration of uterine support. Am J Obstet Gynecol 70:500–513

Almy TP (1977) Therapeutic strategy in stress-related disorders. Clin Gastroenterol 6:709–722

Atlee HB (1966) Acute and chronic iliac pain in women. A problem in diagnosis. Thomas, Springfield Ill

Bond M (1971) The relation of pain to the Eysenck Personality Inventory, Cornell Medical Index and Whiteley Index of hypochondriasis. Br J Psychol 119:671–678

Chapman CR (1978) Pain: the perception of noxious events. In: Sternbach RA (ed) The psychology of pain. Raven Press, New York, pp 169–202

Cotte G (1949) Les troubles fonctionnels de l'appareil génital de la femme. Masson, Paris

Cotte G, Dechaume J (1931) Les plexalgies hypogastriques. Documents histopathologiques. Considérations pathogéniques. Presse Med 39:373

De Brux JA, Bret JA, Demay C, Bardiaux M (1968) Recurring pelvic peritonitis. Am J Obstet Gynecol 102:501–505

Doyle JB (1955) Paracervical uterine denervation by transsection of the cervical plexus for the relief of dysmenorrhea. Am J Obstet Gynecol 70:1–16

Fielding JF (1977) The irritable bowel syndrome, Part I – Clinical spectrum. Clin Gastroenterol 6:607–621

Freund R (1933) Die Krankheiten des Beckenbindegewebes. In: Veit J, Stoeckel W (eds) Handbuch der Gynäkologie, vol VIII, part 1. Bergmann, Leipzig, pp 446–717

Gauss CJ (1949) Eine häufig vorkommende, mehrfach beschriebene, meist verkannte und oft operativ umsonst angegangene Erkrankung: die Pelipathia vegetativa. Dtsch Med Wochenschr 74:1288–1290

Greiss FC, Anderson SG (1970) Effects of ovarian hormones on the uterine vascular bed. Am J Obstet Gynecol 107:829–836

Hathaway JR, Kinley JC (1951) Minnesota multiphasic personality inventory: Manual. The Psychological Corporation, New York

Hein DR, Eskes TKAB, Stolte LAM, Braaksma JT, Janssens J, van den Hoek JM (1972) The influence of steroids on uterine motility in the non-pregnant human uterus. In: Josimovich JB (ed) Uterine contraction – Side effects of steroidal contraceptives. Wiley, New York London, pp 107–128

Jeffcoate N (1975) Textbook of gynaecology, 4th edn. Butterworths, London Boston

Keller B, Wolff F, Leissner P, Swarzberg R, Foegle J (1972) La déchirure du feuillet postérieur du ligament large. Rev Fr Gynecol 67:315–320

Knörr K, Beller FK, Lauritzen C (1972) Lehrbuch der Gynäkologie. Springer, Berlin Heidelberg New York

Koninckx PR, Renaer M, Brosens IA (1980) Origin of peritoneal fluid in women: an ovarian exudation product. Br J Obstet Gynaecol 87:177–183

Lászlo J, Györy G (1959) Histologische Beiträge zum klinischen Bild der „Parametrose". Zentralbl Gynaekol 81:1868–1877

Lászlo J, Györy G (1963) Pathogenesis of pelvic pain. Am J Obstet Gynecol 85:141–148

Louros N (1927) Zur operativen Behandlung der sogenannten Parametritis posterior. Zentralbl Gynaekol 49:3109–3111

Maathuis JB, van Look PFA, Michie EA (1978) Changes in volume, total protein and ovarian steroid concentrations of peritoneal fluid throughout the human menstrual cycle. J Endocrinol 76:123–133

Makowski EL (1977) Vascular physiology. In: Wynn R (ed) Biology of the uterus. Plenum, New York, pp 77–99

Martin E (1944) Die Erkrankungen des Beckenbindegewebes. In: Seitz L, Amreich P (eds) Biologie und Pathologie des Weibes, vol VI. Urban & Schwarzenberg, Wien, pp 1–28

Martius H (1939) Die Kreuzschmerzen der Frau. Thieme, Leipzig

Merskey H (1972) Personality traits of psychiatric patients with pain. J Psychosom Res 16:163–166

Merskey H (1978) Pain and personality. In: Sternbach RA (ed) The psychology of pain. Raven, New York, pp 111–128

Merskey H, Spear FG (1967) Pain. Psychological and psychiatric aspects. Bailliere Tindall & Cassell, London
Mills WG (1978) The enigma of pelvic pain. J R Soc Med 71:257–260
Montgomery JB: see discussion of paper of Stearns and Sneeden (1966)
Neumann HO (1933) Die Krankheiten der Uterusbänder einschließlich Beckenbindegewebe. In: Henke F, Lubarsch O (eds) Handbuch der speziellen pathologischen Anatomie und Histologie, vol VII, part 2. Springer, Berlin, pp 399–622
Novak ER, Jones GS, Jones HW (1975) Novak's textbook of gynecology, 9th edn. Williams & Wilkins, Baltimore
Opitz E (1922) Die Überregbarkeit der glatten Muskulatur der weiblichen Geschlechtsorgane. Zentralbl Gynaekol 40:1594–1598
Parsons L, Sommers SC (1978) Gynecology, 2nd edn. Saunders, Philadelphia
Pilowsky I (1978) Psychodynamic aspects of the pain experience. In: Sternbach RA (ed) The psychology of pain. Raven, New York, pp 203–217
Prill HJ (1964) Psychosomatische Gynäkologie. Urban & Schwarzenberg, München Berlin
Rabkin JG, Struening EL (1976) Life events, stress and illness. Science 194:1013–1020
Renaer M, Vertommen H, Nijs P, Wagemans L, van Hemelrijck T (1979) Psychic aspects of pelvic pain in women. Am J Obstet Gynecol 134:75–80
Renaer M, Nijs P, van Assche A, Vertommen H (1980) Chronic pelvic pain without obvious pathology. Personal observations and a review of the problem. Eur J Obstet Gynecol Reprod Biol 10:415–463
Reynolds SRM (1949) Physiology of the uterus. Hoeber, New York
Schockaert JA (1956) La résection élargie du plexus hypogastrique supérieur et inférieur dans les formes douloureuses de la neurodystonie pelvienne. Bull Soc R Belg Gynecol Obstet 26:174–205
Stearns HC, Sneeden VD (1966) Observations on the clinical and pathological aspects of the pelvic congestion syndrome. Am J Obstet Gynecol 94:718–732
Sternbach RA (1978) Clinical aspects of pain. In: Sternbach RA (ed) The psychology of pain. Raven, New York, pp 241–264
Sternbach RA, Wolf SR, Murphy RW, Akeson WH (1973) Aspects of chronic low back pain. Psychosomatics 14:52–56
Taylor HC (1949 a) Vascular congestion and hyperemia. I. Physiologic basis and history of the concept. Am J Obstet Gynecol 57:211–230
Taylor HC (1949 b) Vascular congestion and hyperemia. II. The clinical aspects of the congestion-fibrosis syndrome. Am J Obstet Gynecol 57:637–653
Taylor HC (1949 c) Vascular congestion and hyperemia. III. Etiology and therapy. Am J Obstet Gynecol 57:654–668
Taylor HC (1961) The syndrome of pelvic pain in women. Aust NZ J Obstet Gynaecol 1:5–16
Theobald GW (1951) Pelvic sympathetic syndrome. J Obstet Gynaecol Br Emp 58:733–761
Truc JB, Musset R (1973) Pathologie du tissu cellulaire pelvien et grossesse. In: De Brux J (ed) Le tissu cellulaire pelvien. Masson, Paris
Vertommen H, Rochette F (1978) Vragenlijst Interpersoonlijke Relaties: V.I.R. Swetz en Zeitlinger, Amsterdam (Interpersonal relations questionnaire V.I.R.)
Wilde GJS (1963) Neurotische labiliteit gemeten volgens de vragenlijstmethode. Van Rossem, Amsterdam
Woodforde JM, Merskey H (1972) Personality traits of patients with chronic pain. J Psychosom Res 16:167–172
Young J (1938) Lower abdominal pains of cervical origin, their genesis and treatment. Br Med J I:104–111
Young J (1947) A textbook of gynaecology. Black, London

19 Treatment of Pain Due to Gynecologic Tumors Localized in the Pelvis (H. Adriaensen and J. Gybels)

19.1 Introduction

The best results of pain relief are obtained when a combination of different methods is made available in a multidisciplinary pain clinic (Bonica 1974). The universal approach with analgesic drugs, as used by every doctor, can often be corrected and improved upon by specialists with a larger pharmacologic experience. At the same time, a pain clinic has facilities for screening patients who would benefit from more specialized intervention.

In this chapter, analgesic drug treatment, nerve blocks, and neurosurgical procedures are discussed as therapeutic modalities for the treatment of pain due to gynecologic tumors localized in the pelvis.

19.2 Treatment of Cancer Pain with Analgesic Drugs

For the therapeutic use of analgesic drugs in cancer pain, the pharmacologic properties of the analgesic drugs must meet the clinical requirements of the patient.

19.2.1 Pharmacologic Properties of Analgesic Drugs

On a pharmacologic basis, the analgesic drugs have for many years been classified as either nonnarcotic or narcotic drugs. More recently, some morphinomimetic compounds with good analgesic potency and low abuse liability have been synthesized, which from a clinical standpoint should be classified as an intermediate group between the minor antiphlogistic agents and the potent narcotics (De Schepper 1975).

The nonnarcotic drugs are supposed to act mainly at the peripheral level, where noxious stimuli cause tissue damage. They block the biosynthesis of the prostaglandines of the E_2 group at the receptor sites (Deraedt et al. 1976; Kuehl and Egan 1977). Besides their analgesic properties, they may show some antiphlogistic and antipyretic activity.

The mechanism of action of the narcotic drugs and their derivatives is situated at the level of the central nervous system. They diminish pain via certain inhibitory systems, which are physiologically activated by endogenous morphine-like substances that act as neurotransmitters (Snyder 1977). Depending on their stereochemical structure, narcotics activate or block a specific morphine receptor. Their activity can be purely agonist or mixed agonist-antagonist.

The choice of analgesic drugs is large. As long as their pharmacologic site of interaction with pain mechanisms is different, two analgesics can be used in combination (Houde et al. 1960). If one drug has competitive or antagonistic properties with the second, their combined use should be avoided (Houde 1974).

19.2.2 Clinical Aspects of Cancer Pain

Analgesic drug treatment is only one way to treat cancer pain. It is a symptomatic treatment and can be complemented by other palliative measures, e. g., neurosurgery, nerve blocks, radiotherapy (Gybels et al. 1976).
Furthermore, it should be kept in mind that pain in patients with advanced cancer must be treated in the context of their terminal illness. Besides their medical care, these patients need human communication. As Gusterson (1977) reported:

> I no longer think that pain relief is the most important feature of our work, except in rare cases . . . It is more important to relieve fear and anxiety, and above all to break down tension between patients and their families. Much of my time is spent listening to patients and their relatives . . .

These aspects are to be taken into account when the results of analgesic drug treatment are evaluated.

19.2.3 Therapeutic Use of Analgesic Drugs

To use analgesic drugs in cancer pain with some efficacy, the analgesic potency and the specific characteristics of the drug administered should match the intensity and nature of the patient's pain.
As far as analgesic potency is concerned, a hierarchic scale can be established on the basis of the clinical results obtained with analgesics. At the bottom of this scale are the aspirin-like drugs and the aspirin combinations; in the middle range, the intermediary group of narcotic derivatives with low addictive properties; and at the top, the potent narcotic agents (Baines 1979).
Depending on the clinical stage of tumor growth, one drug may offer better relief than another. Pain due to a malignant process infiltrating the neighboring tissue sometimes responds to aspirin-like drugs, but often the use of narcotics is necessary. Antiphlogistic analgesics are often successful in pain due to bone metastasis, a process that has been shown to be accompanied by the release of prostaglandins.
Finally, headaches resulting from intracranial hypertension due to brain metastasis may respond well to corticoids. Where nerve tissue has been invaded by the tumor, the pain may be attenuated by tricyclic antidepressants combined with minor analgesics or with narcotics if necessary.

19.2.4 Concomitant Medication

Narcotic medication is often combined with an antiemetic agent of the phenothiazine group. Originally, chlorpromazine (Largactil) was used. This drug has a combined sedative and anxiolytic effect (Kielholz 1972). If sedation has already been achieved by the narcotic medication, it is possible to use prochlorperazine (Stemetil) or domperidone (Motilium).
The analgesic effects of a combination of narcotics and amphetamine-like drugs should be additive (Forrest et al. 1977). Especially in patients who are suscept-

ible to the sedative component of narcotic medication, a single morning dose of dextroamphetamine (Captagon) is rewarding. The amphetamines need not necessarily be used from the beginning of the therapy as the sedative effect of narcotics may wear off after a few days. In pronounced anxiety states, amphetamine medication is contraindicated.

Tricyclic antidepressants show some intrinsic analgesic activity (Kocher 1976) and may be quite effective in denervation pain. They are often used in combination with carbamazepine (Tregretal), an antiepileptic drug, or with aspirin. The psychotropic effect of the drug may improve the mood of the patient. Most authors insist on the use of rather high doses of tricyclic antidepressants for the treatment of pain (Laplane 1979). This may make hospitalization necessary, especially during the first 2 weeks, when their side effects may be rather pronounced. After this period, the patient adapts to the treatment, and the side effects are often less prominent. The most common problems with antidepressant drugs are orthostatic hypotension and states of confusion, especially in the elderly or debilitated patient.

Laxatives will often have to be combined with narcotic analgesics to avoid constipation.

19.2.5 Mode of Administration

Oral administration of analgesics, if possible, should receive priority. Indeed, chronic parenteral medication with analgesics has disadvantages; the patient needs someone to administer the parenteral injection at regular intervals and is made dependent upon this person.

If the patient is not in the hospital, the risk of irregular administration exists. Periods of good pain relief and euphoria (the kick) will then be followed by periods of agony and pain if the injection comes late (Admiraal et al. 1972).

The same oscillations exist when analgesic drugs are administered "on demand." In such a schedule, one can discern the following steps:

- The patient has pain
- The patient complains and asks for analgesic medication
- The medication is given and a state of comfort, perhaps even euphoria, ensues
- Comfort and euphoria, through operant conditioning, positively reinforce a complaining attitude

Thus, medication on demand induces, through its consequences, a more pronounced complaining behavior. When the analgesic medication is given on a time-contigent basis, these reinforcing mechanisms of the complaining behavior are avoided.

Analgesic medication is therefore best given orally, in a preventive way based on a 24-h schedule, in which the intervals between two doses are determined as a function of the duration of the drug's action (Halpern 1974).

19.2.6 Side Effects

Before shifting from one drug to another, because of insufficient pain relief, one should increase the dosage till no further increase in analgesic activity is noticed or until side effects become prominent. At this stage, the drug would offer more discomfort than analgesia so that the use of a stronger drug becomes necessary.

In fact, the main problems in analgesic drug treatment are the side effects: nausea and vomiting, constipation, gastric irritation, dizziness, respiratory depression, and addiction (Vourc'h et al. 1971). These side effects in turn engender other medications: antiemetics, laxatives, antacids, and phenothiazines. Analgesic treatment should always be undertaken with a good deal of suspicion lest the patient become intoxicated by the drugs and suffer from anorexia, sedation, lack of initiative, tiredness, or exhaustion; in extreme cases, the patient may even stop moving. Indirectly, drug intoxication can give rise to nutritional deficiency, respiratory infection, bed sores, depression, and general deterioration.

This condition must be avoided because the patients realize that the medication does harm their general condition and are dissatisfied. Therefore, therapy must be readapted continuously: drugs that are not effective must be canceled; side effects, as they are often transient, must be reevaluated.

In contrast with these real difficulties in the management of chronic analgesic drug therapy, addiction to narcotics is not often the major problem in the treatment of patients with terminal cancer. A difference seems to exist between patients with pain in a disease context and narcotic addicts as a social phenomenon. The evolution from the first to the second group is not mandatory.

Colpaert (1978) was able to demonstrate in animal experiments that rats without pain became tolerant to the analgesic effect of bezitramide, whereas after the experimental induction of a state of chronic pain the same rats showed less tolerance to the analgesic effect of bezitramide. Twycross, who treated cancer patients in St. Christopher's Hospice with diacetylmorphine, noticed a similar phenomenon among his patient population. He did not need to increase the dosage manifestly, even after months of treatment, and for some of them he was even able to decrease it (Twycross and Wald 1976).

If further experimental work should add more evidence to these findings, this might have far-reaching implications for the treatment of chronic pain patients with narcotics.

19.3 Treatment of Cancer Pain with Nerve Blocks

In selected cases in which pain is localized and confined to a restricted area of the body, corresponding to a well-defined innervation, neurolytic blocks may be of some value. In gynecology, cancer pain localized in the pelvis is generally caused by a malignant process of the cervix, the uterus, the ovaries, or the vulva or by metastatic dissemination.

In cancer of the cervix and the uterus, the pain is most often localized in the lower abdomen, the perineum; it may eventually radiate into the lower limbs if

there is extension toward the sacral plexus. Vulvar cancer remains rather well-localized and gives rise to pain in the perineum and the groin.
Cancer of the ovary, often complicated by ascites or subobstruction, gives more diffuse pain over the whole abdomen. Metastatic processes in the skeleton or in the brain result in bone pain or headache. When the pain has remained localized, it may be present on the midline of the body or in an iliac fossa.

19.3.1 Midline Pain

1) *Pain in the lower abdomen and perineal pain* as in cancer of the cervix, the uterus, or the vulva. It is rather difficult to block this pain without affecting the sphincters. If one decides to take this risk, intrathecal phenol, chlorocresol, or alcohol can be used (Swerdlow 1974).
2) *Diffuse abdominal pain* as often present with ovarian cancer. This pain is a complex phenomenon, due to intra-abdominal dissemination, with a tension component of ascites and sometimes abdominal cramps due to subocclusion. No good block procedures exist for this pain, but some relief can be offered by the installation of a Leveen shunt for ascites drainage or by derivative surgery to treat the subobstruction (Leveen et al. 1976).
3) *Generalized metastases* with pain in different parts of the body may be treated with neurolysis of the hypophysis (Moricca 1976).

19.3.2 Unilateral Pain

1) *One-sided pain in the pelvis or groin* or sacral plexus invasion in the early stage can both be treated with intrathecal neurolytics. Nevertheless, percutaneous chordotomy is the treatment of choice for these pain states (Lipton 1974).
2) In the late stage of *nerve tissue invasion,* where some causalgic denervation complicates the clinical picture, blocks or surgical procedures do not seem to be very successful, and tricyclic antidepressants with aspirine-like or narcotic analgesics may offer at least some comfort, although the treatment of this condition remains difficult (Laplane 1979).
3) *Isolated bone metastasis* in the ribs or the vertebrae with unilateral radicular irradiation are suitable for phenol block but are also often alleviated by radiotherapy.

19.4 Neurosurgical Treatment of Cancer Pain of Gynecologic Origin

Carcinomas of gynecologic origin often produce severe pains in the course of their growth. This is related to limited space in the pelvis for tumor expansion, local tumor spread via lymphatics, and proximity to major nerve plexuses. Not only the malignant process itself but also the sequelae of surgery and radiation therapy can lead to pain. In cancer pain, there is obviously tissue damage and,

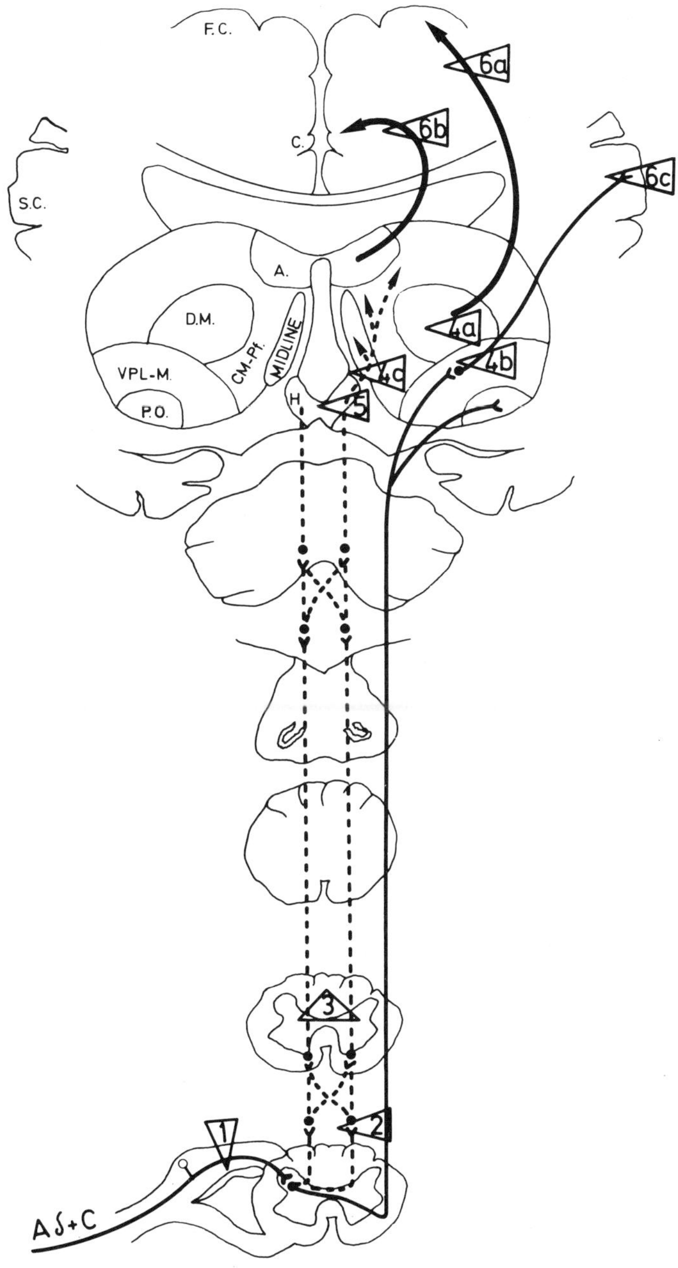

Fig. 22. Abbreviations: —— tractus neospinothalamicus; ---- tractus paleospinothalamicus and spinoreticulothalamicus; → thalamic radiations to frontal cortex and cingulum; *P.O.*, posterior region; *VPL-M,* N. ventralis posterior lateralis and medialis; *D.M.*, N. dorsomedialis; *CM-Pf.*, centrum medianum-parafascicular complex; *MIDLINE,* midline nuclei; *A.*, anterior nuclear group; *H.*, hypothalamus; *F.C.*, frontal cortex; *C.*, cingulum; *S.C.*, somatosensory cortex

therefore, an organic base for the pain complaint is easily found. However, it is obvious that pain complaints in organic disease are not solely a function of noxious input but that there is also a clear-cut relationship between pain and depression and anxiety. Therefore, neurosurgery on its own is usually not sufficient to treat a patient with cancer pain.

Generally speaking, the most favorable candidates for a neurosurgical procedure developed to relieve pain are patients with malignancies that are beyond radiotherapeutic, surgical, or chemical control. This a probably so because the patient's life expectancy is limited and at least part of the pain is due to activation of nociceptors lying in the territory of the cancer process. Although neurosurgical therapy for pain in cancer is often considered a last resort, it is our opinion that it should not be delayed unnecessarily until tolerance to narcotics develops. This is particularly so since new techniques have been developed in the last decade that make old operations safer, easier, and more accurate and new ideas about the neural mechanisms of pain have appeared from which an entirely new form of pain control has evolved: electric stimulation of some neural systems, which may be effective in pain control without destruction of neural tissue.

19.4.1 Lesion Techniques

Lesion techniques are based on classic and more modern notions of the pathways in the nervous system that transmit the information from nociceptors to the higher levels of the nervous system.

These pathways are very complex indeed (for review, see Zimmermann 1976); for our purpose, it is important to observe that there is a lateral and medial afferent system subserving pain (Fig. 22). The lateral pathway that has been described for a long time is composed of the neospinothalamic tract and projects largely contralaterally in a somatotopically organized manner to the somatosen-

Table 10. Neurosurgical techniques

Neurosurgical techniques
Dorsal rhizotomy
Anterolateral cordotomy
Myelotomy
Thalamotomy
Dorsomedial thalamotomy
Ventroposterior thalamotomy (VPM, VPL)
Medial thalamotomy (CM-Pf, intralaminar n.)
Ventroposterior + medial thalamotomy (4b + 4c)
Pulvinarotomy
Hypothalamotomy
Cerebral operations for relief of pain
Frontal leukotomy
Cingulotomy
Postcentral gyrectomy

sory cortex; it is suggested that this pathway conditions the "epicritic" quality of pain. It is only in recent years that knowledge has accumulated concerning the medial pathways. These pathways, composed of paleospinothalamic and spinoreticulothalamic fibers, project diffusely and bilaterally to many subcortical and cortical nonspecific areas. It is suggested that this medial system conditions the "protopathic" quality of pain.

In Table 10, a list is given of the different neurosurgical techniques developed to interrupt these pathways at a certain level. This list is not exhaustive.

It cannot be the purpose of this short review to describe the rationale, indications, and dangers of each of these interventions, and we will limit our discussion to those aspects that are of particular interest to the gynecologist. However, the interested reader can find much information and many references in White and Sweet's monograph (1969) and in Vol. 7 and 8 of *Progress in Neurological Surgery* (Krayenbühl et al. 1976, 1977).

19.4.1.1 Dorsal Rhizotomy

The walls of the pelvic region have their sensory innervation by way of the sacrococcygeal roots; its viscera depend essentially on the presacral sympathetic system (approximately roots D-8–L-2). A major problem with sacral dorsal rhizotomies for pelvic pain is the impairment of urinary and anal sphincters that follow bilateral denervation and, therefore, bilateral sacral rhizotomies are only acceptable for patients who already have urinary and anal sphincter dysfunction. Indeed, the S-2 roots are essential for voiding and the S-3 for defecation. Unilateral rhizotomies are usually well tolerated. If there is pain in the limbs and therefore involvement of segments higher than S-2, dorsal rhizotomy will lead to difficulties with lower limb function. Data on the efficacy of dorsal rhizotomy for visceral and perineal pain due to cancer can be found in Loeser (1979). From an analysis of these data, it appears that dorsal rhizotomy can be useful only in certain localized forms of painful pelvic cancers.

19.4.1.2 Anterolateral Cordotomy

Section of the anterolateral quadrant of the spinal cord is one of the oldest neurosurgical operations for pain relief. This operation can provide a selective loss of pain and temperature sensation in a widespread region of the body without an impairment of other sensory modalities. A percutaneous technique, introduced about a decade ago (Mullan et al. 1963) in which an electrode is introduced into the anterolateral quadrant of the spinal cord, has many advantages: no incision is necessary, no general anesthesia is required, pathways can be identified in the conscious cooperative patient by electrophysiologic techniques, and lesions can be placed in a sufficiently precise manner. It follows that the indication for cordotomy can now be extended to those patients who are too ill for an open procedure and that complications, such as death, paralysis, and sphincter impairment, can be reduced.

Not infrequently, a patient who reports unilateral pain will after a cordotomy complain of pain at the previously nonpainful side. This is possibly due to a masking of the minor pain by the more severe one. When the major one is relieved, the minor one is recognized.

Midline pain requires bilateral cordotomy for adequate relief. In that case, a high risk remains of bladder dysfunction. A rather important, but avoidable complication, seen with high cordotomies, is related to respiration: when this complication arises, the patient breathes normally when awake but becomes apneic when asleep. The complication is due to the interruption of an ascending system mediated through the upper cervical cord in the white matter immediately adjacent to the anterior horn and which contributes to the control of ventilation. This complication can, according to Rosomoff et al. (1969), be predicted by testing the patient for his response to breathing carbon dioxide.

Recent data on the efficacy of anterolateral cordotomy for visceral and perineal pain due to cancer are given in Loeser (1979). They show that cordotomy is a particularly effective surgical therapy for visceral and perineal pain due to cancer.

19.4.1.3 Myelotomy

Lumbosacral myelotomy (commissurotomy, mediolongitudinal myelotomy) is an ancient and well-established procedure. It was originally designed to divide the decussating fibers of the spinothalamic pathway to treat bilateral cancer body pain. Wertheimer and Sautot (1949), reporting the results in 59 cases of thoracic commissurotomies, produced anesthetic areas in only 23 patients, and yet they produced total pain relief in 29 and a failure in only 13 cases. In their opinion, therefore, the results of pain relief could not be correlated with the presence or absence of changes in temperature or pain sensations.

We now know that the pain relief observed in this operation may be due to an interruption of the multisynaptic, diffusely projecting medial paleospinothalamic and spinoreticulothalamic fiber systems that conduct nociceptive input.

Since Hitchcock (1970) introduced stereotactic cervical myelotomy, the interruption of the medial nociceptive input systems has become easier, and since then this operation has been gaining in popularity (Schvarcz 1976). This stereotactic method has indeed many advantages over conventional myelotomy. It is a much less traumatic intervention than open myelotomy, it can be applied without problem to the awake patient, the accuracy of the electrode placement can be checked by stimulation, and the extent of the lesion monitored by noting neurologic signs and more specifically the degree of analgesia produced. There are not enough data available as yet to permit a sufficiently precise evaluation of this operation in pelvic cancer pain.

19.4.1.4 Thalamotomy

Although about 30 years have passed since Spiegel and Wycis (1953) performed the first stereotactic procedure on the human thalamus for relief of pain and although thalamotomy has been by far the most widely used stereotactic procedure for pain relief, it is still difficult to formulate guidelines for patient and target selection and to make a realistic prognosis. Three physiologic systems in the thalamus have been used as stereotactic therapeutic targets:

1) The projection of the spinothalamic and quintothalamic tracts in the basal part of the specific relay nuclei VPM-VPL
2) The nonspecific polysynaptic system with the intralaminar nuclei and their adjacent fibers
3) The frontothalamic system with the dorsomedial and anterior group of nuclei

The two first systems probably are more concerned with the discriminative aspects of pain, while the third is more concerned with the affective aspects of pain. Finally, although almost nothing is known about its function in nociception, lesions are also placed in the pulvinar for pain control (Siegfried 1977).

Recently, Tasker (to be published) made an extensive and critical review of the results of stereotactic thalamic surgery for pain. In evaluating results, he distinguishes between (1) "somatic" pain, where the noxious stimulus is detected by nociceptors and transmitted over pain fibers to the dorsal horns and relayed over the spinothalamic and spinoreticular system to appropriate nuclei in the brainstem and thalamus and (2) "dysesthetic" pain, where the sensation is not conditioned by activation of nociceptors but due to central perturbation, caused by deafferentation. Tasker states further that cancer commonly causes somatic pain by tissue stretch, inflammation, and chemical stimuli but also dysesthetic pain through destruction of nerve elements.

According to Tasker's review, in summarizing the results of thalamotomy for pain, one is struck by the fact that two-thirds of patients with somatic pain have enjoyed good results with lesions in widely scattered areas of the thalamus. Lesions made in the specific pain relays or in the pulvinar appear most successful. For the patient with dysesthetic pain, however, the results are far less promising, and satisfactory relief was reported only in about 25% of the patients, no matter where the lesion was placed. Despite these rather dissatisfying results, stereotactic thalamotomy remains a possibility in patients with uncontrolled pelvic pain.

19.4.1.5 Hypothalamotomy

Although only a few neurosurgeons – and only recently (Fairman 1973) – have reported on favorable results in cancer pain after medial posterior hypothalamotomy and obviously this intervention at the moment should be restricted to a very few neurosurgical centers, we refer to this intervention here because those favorable results may give a clue to the understanding of the surprisingly favorable results reported after chemical hypophysectomy by Moricca (1976) and this as well in non-hormone-dependent as in hormone-dependent neoplastic disease. This author injects through needles placed in the sella tursica by way of the nose 0.6–2 ml ethanol. According to Moricca, pituitary adenolysis constitutes a nontraumatic and easily performed technique: it does not require special equipment, is absolutely inexpensive, and can be repeated without any technical limitations and with insignificant clinical contraindications. It controls with a single block diffuse, unbearable cancer pain. Up to 1975, he treated 1026 patients with advanced malignancy, performing 2372 pituitary chemolyses. The treatment was carried out mostly in patients with visceral and bone-associated metastases. Most of these patients were in very poor condition; they all suffered from diffuse and severe cancer pain. In 885 cases, pain relief was complete, immediate, and long-lasting. These results, if they are true, are very impressive indeed. They need, of course, confirmation and proper evaluation by others, but at a first glance would point to chemical hypophysectomy as a unique method for relieving "unbearable" cancer pain.

At this point, one may ask what could be the mechanisms through which chemical hypophysectomy produces its antalgic actions, and particularly so in the case of the non-hormone-dependent cancer disease. A possible explanation is the observation made by Miles and Lipton (1976), who showed that fluids injected into the pituitary gland propagate through the pituitary stalk and into the region of the hypothalamus; consequently, pain relief in chemical hypophysectomy might be due to chemical hypothalamotomy.

19.4.1.6 Cerebral Operations

For a long time, frontal leukotomy and cingulotomy have been employed as a last resort to attenuate the psychic and emotional experience of pain. Well-known and rarely used nowadays, they need not be discussed here. Gyrectomy of the somesthetic cortical area is not effective and has been abandoned.

19.4.2 Stimulation Techniques

The publication in 1965 of the gate theory of pain perception by Melzack and Wall and the discovery, mainly by Mayer et al. (1971), of a medial brainstem system with the specific and apparently endogenous property of pain inhibition has led to a renewed interest in the use of electric stimulation of neural systems for pain relief. Although today not many clinical data are available on this form of treatment in cancer pain of pelvic origin, the theoretical implications and the possible clinical applications are of such importance that they should be briefly discussed here. Important information on this topic can be found in recent reviews (Sedan and Lazorthes 1978; Albe-Fessard and Gybels 1979).

19.4.2.1 Dorsal Column Stimulation

Schematically, dorsal column stimulation is performed by implanting electrodes on the dorsal column. These electrodes are connected to a miniature radiofrequency receiver, which is implanted under the skin, usually in the thoracic region under the clavicula. Electric stimulation is supplied by a miniature battery-powered radio transmitter that produces a square wave of variable frequency, voltage, and pulse width, which is coupled to the receiver by the use of a flexible antenna. The patient chooses those parameters with which the best pain relief is experienced.

Dorsal column stimulation has as physiologic background that according to the gate theory, nociceptive input, which is conducted to the central nervous system via small fibers (Van Hees and Gybels 1972), can be inhibited by activation of the large fiber somatic afferent system.

Dorsal column stimulation has been employed in thousands of patients with all kinds of pains. Initial results appeared quite promising with over 80% of patients describing pain relief. With time, this percentage has steadily fallen. It now appears that in the most carefully selected series, a success rate of about 50% is to be expected (Long and Hagfors 1975). As far as cancer pain is concerned, no precise data are as yet available in the literature, but it seems that dorsal column stimulation poorly controls cancer pain of visceral origin.

19.4.2.2 Brain Stimulation

It is now well-known that electric stimulation of periaqueductal and periventricular gray has a potent analgesic effect in acute pain in animals (Mayer et al. 1971), probably by activating an endogenous "opiate" system. Since the first publications (Richardson and Akil 1977) reporting that intractable clinical pain states in humans, in addition to normal pain perception, can be blocked by electric stimulation of periaqueductal and periventricular gray matter, a European study group collected in 1979 data on 143 cases (European Workshop 1979). It appeared from this cooperative study that success was somewhat less than 50% and that cancer pain responded better to this stimulation than the other types of pain. Although it is still to early to evaluate with accuracy (Gybels 1979) the usefulness of this stimulation, in contradiction to dorsal column stimulation, it seems to be most effective in cancer pain, and theoretically well-suited for the difficult-to-treat midline or bilaterally distributed pain as seen in cancer pain of gynecologic origin.

A large number of procedures to relieve cancer pain of gynecologic origin are available. The choice of a procedure will depend on the problems, proper to each individual patient, and the experience a particular neurosurgeon has with a given procedure. All methods used for the treatment of pain have their shortcomings, however (for review, see Gybels et al. 1976), and the neurosurgical techniques we have outlined here are no exception to this rule.

19.5 Conclusion

Three modalities for the treatment of cancer pain in gynecology are reviewed. The discussion is not exhaustive, and other approaches, e. g., psychotherapy, palliative radiotherapy, and chemotherapy, may broaden the therapy. It cannot be overemphasized, however, that to treat well, insight is required not only in the available therapeutic procedures, but also in the clinical condition of the patient with pain.

References

Admiraal PV, Knape H, Zegveld C (1972) Experience with bezitramide and droperidol in the treatment of severe chronic pain. Br J Anaesth 44:1191–1196

Albe-Fessard D, Gybels J (1979) La douleur. Rapports présentés au XLIIe Congrès Français de Médecine, Liège, 1979. Masson, Paris, p 129

Baines M (1979) Médications symptomatiques les plus courantes dans les états terminaux. Rev Prat 29:1619–1626

Bonica JJ (1974) Pain. Adv Neurol 4:850

Colpaert FC (1978) Long term suppression of pain by narcotic drugs in the absence of tolerance development. Arch Int Pharmacodyn Ther 236:293–295

Deraedt R, Jouquey S, Benzoni J, Peterfalvi M (1976) Inhibition of prostaglandine biosynthesis by non-narcotic analgesic drugs. Arch Int Pharmacodyn Ther 224:30–42

De Schepper P (1975) Farmakotherapeutische beschouwingen bij enkele analgetika van het morfinetype: d-propoxypheen, tilidine, pentazocine. Folia Farmakother 2:81–88

European study on deep brain stimulation (1979) Resume of the 3rd European Workshop on Electrical Neurostimulation. Mégève, March 30–31 p 58

Fairman D (1973) Stereotactic hypothalamotomy for the alleviation of pain in malignant tumors. J Surg Oncol 5:79–84

Forrest WH, Brown BW, Brown CR, Defalque R, Gold M, Gordon HE, James KE, Katz J, Mahler DL, Schroff P, Teutsch G (1977) Dextroamphetamine with morphine for the treatment of postoperative pain. N Engl J Med 296/3:712–715

Gusterson FR (1977) Role of residential care in terminal illness. In: Harcus AW, Smith R, Whittle B (eds) Pain: new perspectives in measurement and management. Churchill Livingstone, London, pp 134–137

Gybels J (1979) Electrical stimulation of the central gray for pain relief in humans: a critical review. In: Bonica JJ, Albe-Fessard D, Liebeskind J (eds). Advances in pain research and therapy, vol 3. Raven, New York, pp 499–509

Gybels J, Adriaensen H, Cosyns P (1976) Treatment of pain in patients with advanced cancer. Eur J Cancer 12:341–351

Halpern LM (1974) Psychotropic drugs and the management of chronic pain. Adv Neurol 4:539–545

Hitchcock E (1970) Stereotactic cervical myelotomy. J Neurol Neurosurg Psychiatry 33:224–230

Houde RW (1974) The use and misuse of narcotics in the treatment of chronic pain. Adv Neurol 4:527–536

Houde RW, Wallenstein MS, Ada Rogers RN (1960) Clinical pharmacology of analgesics: a method of assaying analgesic effect. Clin Pharmacol Ther 1:163–175

Kielholz P (1972) Diagnosis and treatment of psychogenic pain. In: Janzen R, Keidel WD, Herz A, Steichele C (eds) Pain: basic principles – pharmacology – therapy. Churchill Livingstone, London, pp 172–174

Kocher R (1976) The use of psychotropic drugs in the treatment of chronic, severe pain. Eur Neurol 14:458–464

Krayenbühl H, Maspes PE, Sweet WH (eds) (1976) Pain – Its neurosurgical management. Part I: Procedures on primary afferent neurons. Prog Neurol Surg 7:265

Krayenbühl H, Maspes PE, Sweet WH (eds) (1977) Pain – Its neurosurgical management. Part II: Central procedures. Prog Neurol Surg 8:284

Kuehl FA, Egan RW (1977) Prostaglandins and related mediators in pain. In: Miehlke K (ed) Diflunisal in clinical practice. Futura, New York, pp 13–20
Laplane D (1979) L'utilisation des tricycliques comme antalgiques. Rev Prat 29:1593–1599
Leveen HH, Wapnick S, Grosberg S, Kinney MJ (1976) Further experience with peritoneo-venous shunt for ascites. Ann Surg 184:574–580
Lipton S (1974) Percutaneous cervical cordotomy and pituitary injection of alcohol. In: Swerdlow M (ed) Relief of intractable pain. Excerpta Medica, Amsterdam (Monographs in anaesthesiology, vol 1, pp 211–244)
Loeser JD (1979) Role of neurosurgery in visceral and perineal pain. In: Bonica JJ, and Ventafridda V (eds) Advances in pain research and therapy, vol 2. Raven, New York, pp 607–614
Long DM, Hagfors N (1975) Electrical stimulation in the nervous system: the current status of electrical stimulation of the nervous system for relief of pain. Pain 1:109–123
Mayer DJ, Wolfle TL, Akil H, Carder B, Liebeskind JC (1971) Analgesia from electrical stimulation in the brainstem of the rat. Science 174:1351–1354
Melzack R, Wall PD (1965) Pain mechanisms: A new theory. Science 150:971–978
Miles J, Lipton S (1976) The mode of action by which pituitary alcohol injection relieves pain. In: Bonica JJ, Albe-Fessard D (eds) Advances in pain research and therapy, vol 1. Raven, New York, pp 867–869
Moricca G (1976) Neuroadenolystic, chemical hypophysectomy, for diffuse unbearable cancer pain. In: Bonica JJ, Albe-Fessard D (eds) Advances in pain research and therapy, vol 1. Raven, New York, pp 863–866
Mullan S, Harper PV, Hekmatpanah J, Torres H, Dobben G (1963) Percutaneous interruption of spinal-pain tracts by means of a strontium-90 needle. J Neurosurg 20:931–939
Richardson DE, Akil H (1977) Pain reduction by electrical brain stimulation in man. Part 2: Chronic self-administration in the periventricular gray matter. J Neurosurg 47:184–194
Rosomoff HL, Krieger AJ, Kuperman AS (1969) Effects of percutaneous cervical cordotomy on pulmonary function. J Neurosurg 31:620–627
Schvarcz JR (1976) Stereotactic extralemniscal myelotomy. J Neurol Neurosurg Psychiatry 39:53–57
Sedan R, Lazorthes Y (1978) La neurostimulation électrique thérapeutique. Neurochirurgie [Suppl 1] 24:1–138
Siegfried J (1977) Stereotactic pulvinarotomy in the treatment of intractable pain. Prog Neurol Surg 8:104–113
Snyder SH (1977) Opiate receptors and internal opiates. Sci Am 236:42–47
Spiegel EA, Wycis HT (1953) Mesencephalotomy in treatment of intractable facial pain. AMA Arch Neurol Psychiatry 69:1–18
Swerdlow M (1974) Intrathecal and extradural block in pain relief. In: Swerdlow M (ed) Relief of intractable pain. Excerpta Medica, Amsterdam (Monographs in anaesthesiology, vol 1, pp 121–155)
Tasker RR (to be published) Pain: Thalamic procedures. Textbook of stereotaxy of the human brain, 3rd edn. Thieme, Stuttgart
Twycross RG, Wald SJ (1976) Long-term use of diamorphine in advanced cancer. In: Bonica JJ, Albe-Fessard D (eds) Advances in pain research and therapy, vol 1. Raven, New York, pp 653–661
Van Hees J, Gybels J (1972) Pain related to single afferent C fibers from human skin. Brain Res 48:397–400
Vourc'h G, de Castro J, Gauthier-Lafaye P, Giudicelli JF, Viars P (eds) (1971) Principaux analgésiques centraux utilisés en clinique. In: Les analgésiques et la douleur.

Ed: Masson, Cie, Société Francais de Anesthésie, d'Analgésie et de Réanimation, Paris, pp 234–282
Wertheimer P, Sautot J (1949) Les résultats de la myélotomie commissurale postérieure (à propos de 69 observations). Concours Med 71:413–414
White JC, Sweet WH (1969) Pain and the neurosurgeon. Thomas, Springfield, p 1000
Zimmermann M (1976) Neurophysiology of nociception. In: Porter R (ed) International review of physiology, neurophysiology II, vol 10. University Park Press, Baltimore, pp 179–221

Subject Index

Functional Morphologic Changes in Female Sex Organs Induced by Exogenous Hormones

Editor: G. Dallenbach-Hellweg
1980. 139 figures, 42 tables. XV, 234 pages
ISBN 3-540-09885-2

H. Ludwig, H. Metzger

The Human Female Reproductive Tract

A Scanning Electron Microscopic Atlas
1976. 546 micrographs. XI, 247 pages
ISBN 3-540-07675-1

B. J. Masterson

Manual of Gynecologic Surgery

Illustrator: D. McKeown
With contributions by K. E. Krantz, W. J. Cameron, J. W. Daly, J. A. Fayez, E. W. Franklin
1979. 204 figures, 192 in color, 12 tables. XV, 256 pages
(Comprehensive Manuals of Surgical Specialties)
ISBN 3-540-90372-0

Pathology of the Female Genital Tract

Editor: A. Blaustein
1977. 1206 figures, 39 four-color figures. XX, 897 pages
ISBN 3-540-90180-9

N. Hassani

Ultrasonography of the Abdomen

With a contribution by R. Bard
1976. 215 figures. XVI, 127 pages
ISBN 3-540-90166-3

Springer-Verlag
Berlin
Heidelberg
New York